BLOOD TYPE A

DIET COOKBOOK

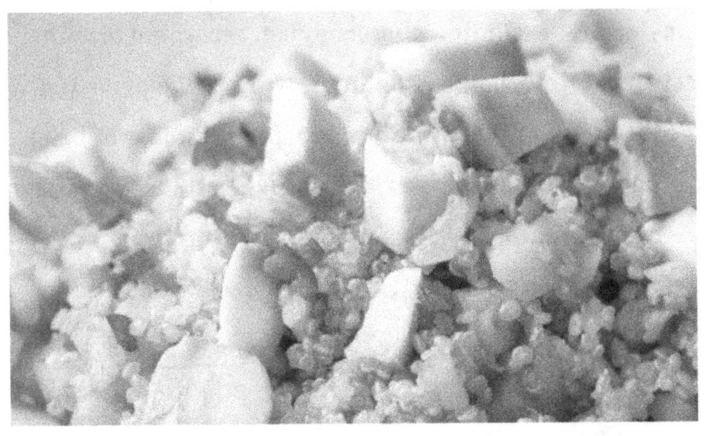

A Comprehensive Guide Featuring Healthy Type A Friendly Recipes for Optimal Health and Wellness

LENA R. FOSTER

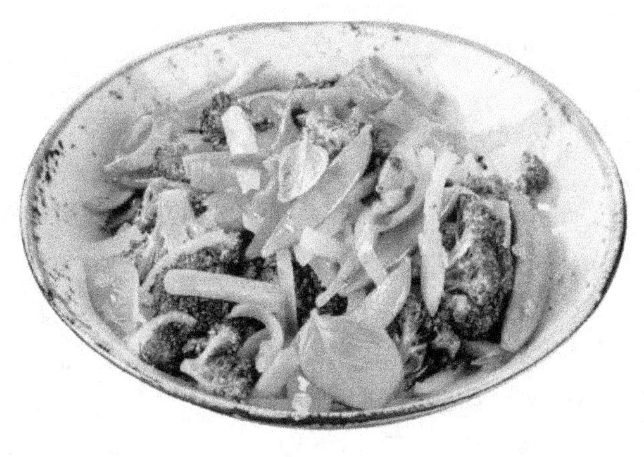

BLOOD TYPE A

DIET COOKBOOK

Table of Contents

INTRODUCTION..8
CHAPTER 1: UNDERSTANDING BLOOD TYPE A........10
BENEFITS OF FOLLOWING BLOOD TYPE A DIET. 12
FOODS TO EAT AND FOODS TO AVOID.................. 14
SHOPPING LIST FOR BLOOD TYPE A DIET.......... 15
TIPS FOR BLOOD TYPE A DIET...............................17
CHAPTER 2: 30-DAY MEAL PLAN................................20
CHAPTER 3: BREAKFAST... 30
Avocado and Spinach Omelet.................................. 30
Sweet Potato Breakfast Hash..................................31
Greek Yogurt Parfait... 32
Egg and Veggie Breakfast Muffins...........................34
Almond Butter Banana Toast...................................35
Millet Breakfast Porridge...36
Green Smoothie Bowl...37
Coconut Chia Pudding..38
Turmeric Scrambled Eggs with Sautéed Greens........39
Quinoa and Berry Breakfast Bowl............................40
Mushroom and Spinach Breakfast Wrap....................41
Buckwheat Pancakes with Mixed Berry Compote...... 43
Chia Seed Pudding with Citrus Infusion.................. 44
Mango-Coconut Overnight Oats................................45
Lentil and Vegetable Breakfast Skillet...................... 47
Tofu Scramble with Spinach and Tomatoes...............48
Buckwheat Banana Pancakes...................................49
Millet Breakfast Bowl with Almond Butter and Berries 50

Avocado and Smoked Salmon Rice Cakes................. 51

CHAPTER 4: LUNCH...54

Lentil and Vegetable Stir-Fry...................................... 54

Chickpea and Avocado Salad....................................56

Salmon and Quinoa Bowl with Lemon-Dill Dressing.. 57

Turkey and Vegetable Lettuce Wraps.......................59

Mediterranean Chickpea Salad................................. 60

Sesame Ginger Tofu Stir-Fry.................................... 61

Quinoa and Vegetable Stuffed Bell Peppers.............63

Eggplant and Chickpea Buddha Bowl....................... 64

Turkey and Vegetable Skillet with Quinoa................. 66

Salmon and Asparagus Foil Packets.........................67

Quinoa and Kale Stuffed Bell Peppers...................... 69

Mushroom and Spinach Quiche................................ 70

Turkey and Sweet Potato Hash................................. 71

Greek Chicken Salad Wrap...................................... 73

Vegetarian Quinoa and Black Bean Bowl..................74

Caprese Chickpea Salad.. 75

Miso-Glazed Salmon Salad...................................... 76

Sweet Potato and Lentil Buddha Bowl.......................78

Spinach and Feta Stuffed Turkey Burgers.................79

Turmeric Chicken and Vegetable Skewers................ 80

CHAPTER 5: SNACKS AND DESSERTS....................82

Baked Kale Chips.. 82

Avocado and Tomato Rice Cakes..............................83

Cucumber and Hummus Bites................................... 84

Egg and Avocado Rice Cake Stack...........................85

Nut Butter Energy Balls... 86

Apple and Almond Butter Slices................................ 87

Carrot and Hummus Roll-Ups...................................88

Tuna and Avocado Cucumber Bites..........................89

Stuffed Bell Pepper Rings.......................................90

Cucumber and Smoked Salmon Roll-Ups.................91

Sweet Potato and Almond Butter Bites.....................92

Cherry Tomato and Goat Cheese Stuffed Celery Sticks. 92

Pomegranate and Cottage Cheese Parfait.................93

Cinnamon Baked Pears...94

Cocoa-Coconut Energy Bites....................................95

Baked Apple Slices with Almond Date Crumble........96

Vanilla Coconut Chia Pudding..................................97

Pistachio Banana Ice Cream....................................98

Maple Pecan Baked Apples......................................99

Cinnamon Pear Yogurt Parfait................................. 100

CHAPTER 6: DINNER.. **102**

Lemon Herb Baked Chicken.................................... 102

Vegetarian Lentil and Sweet Potato Curry................ 103

Zucchini Noodles with Pesto and Cherry Tomatoes. 105

Baked Lemon Garlic Herb Chicken Thighs............... 106

Eggplant and Chickpea Curry................................... 107

Lemon Herb Baked Cod.. 108

Chickpea and Vegetable Curry................................. 109

Mediterranean Quinoa Salad with Grilled Chicken....111

Salmon and Vegetable Foil Packets......................... 112

Stir-Fried Tofu with Broccoli and Cashews............... 113

Lemon Garlic Shrimp with Quinoa........................... 115

Grilled Turkey and Vegetable Skewers..................... 116

Vegetarian Lentil and Spinach Stuffed Bell Peppers. 117

Turkey Stir-Fry with Bok Choy and Brown Rice Noodles 119

Eggplant Lasagna with Ground Turkey and Tomato-Based Sauce.. 121

Turkey Chili with Kidney Beans, Tomatoes, and a Variety of Spices.. 123

Grilled Portobello Mushrooms with Quinoa and Vegetable Stuffing.. 125

CHAPTER 7: SOUPS AND STEWS........................ 128

Quinoa and Kale Soup....................................128

Mushroom and Barley Soup........................... 129

Coconut Chickpea Stew................................. 131

Red Lentil and Spinach Soup......................... 132

Vegetable and Lentil Stew............................. 133

Butternut Squash and Apple Soup.................. 135

Cauliflower and Leek Soup.............................136

Chickpea and Spinach Stew...........................137

Lentil and Vegetable Soup..............................138

Mushroom and Wild Rice Soup...................... 140

Turmeric Cauliflower Soup..............................141

Bean and Kale Sausage Stew........................ 143

CHAPTER 8: SALADS..................................... 146

Quinoa and Chickpea Salad........................... 146

Spinach and Strawberry Salad with Almond Vinaigrette. 147

Mango Avocado Quinoa Salad........................ 149

Greek Lentil Salad... 150

Citrus Avocado Salad..................................... 151

Apple Walnut Quinoa Salad............................152

Asian-Inspired Sesame Ginger Salad..............154

Roasted Beet and Goat Cheese Salad.....................155

Pomegranate and Almond Spinach Salad...............156

Quinoa and Roasted Vegetable Salad.....................158

Cucumber and Chickpea Salad with Lemon Herb Dressing.....................159

CHAPTER 9: SMOOTHIES.....................162

Citrus Avocado Smoothie.....................162

Turmeric Pineapple Bliss Smoothie.....................163

Berry Almond Protein Smoothie.....................164

Coconut Kale Green Smoothie.....................165

Minty Melon Cucumber Smoothie.....................166

Pomegranate Ginger Citrus Smoothie.....................167

Berry Basil Bliss Smoothie.....................168

Coconut Pineapple Kale Smoothie.....................168

Mango Turmeric Sunshine Smoothie.....................169

Blueberry Mint Refresher Smoothie.....................170

Kiwi Basil Bliss Smoothie.....................171

Mango Mint Marvel Smoothie.....................172

Pineapple Kale Harmony Smoothie.....................173

CONCLUSION.....................174

TYPE A DIET WEEKLY MEAL PLAN.....................176

INTRODUCTION

Kelly, who has Blood Type A, began on a revolutionary quest to live a healthy lifestyle. Armed with a Blood Type A Diet Cookbook, she found a world of healthful and tasty meals matched to her blood type.

Kelly began each morning with a colorful meal of leafy greens, tofu, and a cup of green tea. The cookbook helped her make conscientious decisions, emphasizing meals that were compatible with her blood type. As a consequence, she felt invigorated and focused all day.

Lunches were colorful affairs, with a variety of veggies, lean meats, and cereals carefully chosen from the cookbook's suggestions. Kelly's increased cooking talents enabled her to eat meals that not only delighted her palate but also improved her overall health.

Kelly turned dinner into an occasion for culinary discovery as she tried out the cookbook's many dishes. From stir-fried veggies to quinoa salads, each food was painstakingly designed to meet her Blood Type A needs.

The cookbook not only included recipes, but it also educated Kelly on the science of the Blood Type A diet. She understood how particular meals affect her body, and this knowledge enabled her to make educated decisions outside of the kitchen.

Kelly's friends and family saw the good change over the course of many weeks. Her gorgeous skin, better digestion, and robust energy demonstrated the effectiveness of a tailored diet. Kelly had found the Blood Type A Diet Cookbook to be an essential resource on her path to a better and more satisfying life.

Welcome to this Blood Type A Diet Cookbook, your culinary guide to maximum health. In this comprehensive collection of dishes, we welcome you on a trip designed exclusively for those with Blood Type A. Based on the Blood Type Diet's principles, this cookbook will lead you to a better, more harmonious living via the transforming power of individualized nutrition.

CHAPTER 1: UNDERSTANDING BLOOD TYPE A

Blood type A is one of four major blood types, defined by the presence or absence of particular antigens and antibodies in the blood. These antigens and antibodies determine compatibility with blood transfusions and organ transplants.

Here's a full explanation of blood type A:

Genetic Basis:

- Blood type A is identified by the presence of A antigens on the surface of red blood cells.
- It is passed on from parents, with variations determined by genetic factors.

Antigens and Antibodies:

- Individuals with blood type A have both A antigens and anti-B antibodies.
- Anti-B antibodies indicate that people may respond adversely to blood from type B or AB donors.

Medical Significance:

- Important for blood transfusions: Type A persons may get blood from A or O donors.

- Relevant for organ transplants, since matching blood types lowers the chance of rejection.

Health Implications:
- According to certain research, blood type A is associated with a higher risk of certain health issues such as heart disease and cancer.
- Nutritional considerations: A balanced, plant-based diet may be good for those with blood type A.

Cultural Beliefs:
- In certain cultures, blood types are believed to impact personality and compatibility.
- Despite the minimal scientific evidence, these cultural beliefs add an intriguing layer to the relevance of blood kinds.

Compatibility and Transfusions:
- Compatible with blood of type A and O donors.
- Anti-B antibodies make the blood incompatible with those of type B or AB donors.

Research and Evolution of Understanding:

- Ongoing study may reveal more about the link between blood type A and numerous health aspects.
- Advancements in genetic studies contribute to a deeper understanding of blood type variations.

Blood Types and Reproduction:

- Consideration of blood type compatibility in family planning and potential genetic disorders.

Practical Considerations:

- Individuals with blood type A are advised to know their blood type in case of a medical emergency.
- Understanding the health concerns connected with blood type A might help you make preventive healthcare decisions.

BENEFITS OF FOLLOWING BLOOD TYPE A DIET

1. Improved Digestion: Eating a diet tailored to blood type A may lead to improved digestion and nutrient absorption, hence improving overall digestive health.

2. Weight Management: The diet emphasizes plant-based foods, implying that people with blood type A may find it easier to maintain a healthy weight if they avoid some animal products and concentrate on fruits, vegetables, and whole grains.

3. Reduced Inflammation: Eating the suggested foods for blood type A may help decrease inflammation in the body, thereby decreasing the risk of chronic illnesses related with inflammation.

4. Enhanced Immune System: According to the diet, eating certain foods may help to strengthen the immune system, possibly increasing the body's capacity to fight infections and diseases.

5. Increased Energy Levels: Individuals feel more energetic aligning their food choices with the anticipated features of Blood Type A. Diet high in fruits, vegetables, and lean proteins, all of which are usually thought to be good for your health.

6. Balanced Hormones: Eating a diet based on blood type A may help with hormonal balance, perhaps relieving symptoms associated with hormonal imbalances.

FOODS TO EAT AND FOODS TO AVOID

FOODS TO EAT

1. Plant-Based Proteins: Tofu, tempeh, lentils, and beans are good sources of protein for those with blood type A.

2. Whole Grains: Choose grains like quinoa, brown rice, and oats for sustained energy and critical minerals.

3. Fruits and Vegetables: Choose a range of colorful fruits and vegetables that are high in antioxidants and vitamins.

4. Nuts and seeds: Almonds, walnuts, flaxseeds, and pumpkin seeds are good sources of healthful fats and nutrients.

5. Certain Dairy Products: Fermented dairy, such as yogurt, and tiny quantities of goat or sheep milk are often recommended.

6. Green Tea: Advocates advocate green tea for its possible health advantages and antioxidant levels.

FOODS TO AVOID

1. Red Meat: Individuals with blood type A are expected to minimize or avoid red meat owing to probable stomach issues.

2. Certain Dairy Products: Cow's milk and its derivatives are typically avoided because they may be incompatible with blood type A.

3. High-Fat Animal Products: Fatty meat, bacon, and processed meats are normally avoided.

4. Wheat and gluten: Some variants of the diet include limiting wheat and gluten-containing foods.

5. Certain Legumes: While legumes are usually acceptable, certain kinds, such as kidney beans, should be avoided for blood type A.

6. Processed and Highly Refined Foods: Processed and highly refined meals should be avoided for overall health concerns.

SHOPPING LIST FOR BLOOD TYPE A DIET

Proteins
- Tofu
- Tempeh
- Lentils
- Chickpeas
- Black beans
- Navy beans

Whole Grains

- Quinoa
- Brown rice
- Oats
- Buckwheat
- Millet

Fruits

- Blueberries
- Cherries
- Pineapple
- Plums
- Apples
- Berries (strawberries, raspberries)

Vegetables

- Kale
- Spinach
- Broccoli
- Carrots
- Sweet potatoes
- Artichokes

Nuts and Seeds

- Almonds
- Walnuts
- Flaxseeds
- Pumpkin seeds
- Sunflower seeds

Dairy (Limited)

- Goat cheese
- Sheep milk yogurt

Beverages

- Green tea
- Herbal teas
- Water (Stay hydrated)

TIPS FOR BLOOD TYPE A DIET

1. Focus on Fresh and Organic: When feasible, choose fresh, organic vegetables to increase nutritional intake while reducing pesticide exposure.
2. Diversify Your Plate: Choose a variety of colors and varieties of fruits and vegetables to provide a wide range of nutrients.

3. Mindful Protein Choices: Choose plant-based protein sources over red meat. Fish, turkey, and chicken are all regarded as appropriate in moderation.

4. Whole Grains Matter: Whole grains, such as quinoa and brown rice, are important for providing long-term energy and critical minerals.

5. Hydration is essential: Drink enough water throughout the day to keep hydrated and promote overall health.

6. Balanced Meals: To maintain consistent energy levels, aim for balanced meals that contain a variety of protein, healthy fats, and carbs.

7. Experiment with Herbs and Spices: To enhance taste without using too much salt, use herbs and spices such as turmeric, ginger, and basil into your meals.

8. Read Food Labels: Be aware of food labels, particularly when purchasing processed or packaged goods, to prevent undesirable additions and substances.

9. Meal Preparation: Plan and prepare meals ahead of time to prevent eating unhealthy foods when stressed for time.

10. Listen to Your Body: Pay attention to how your body reacts to various meals. Individual reactions vary, so tailor your diet to your individual health.

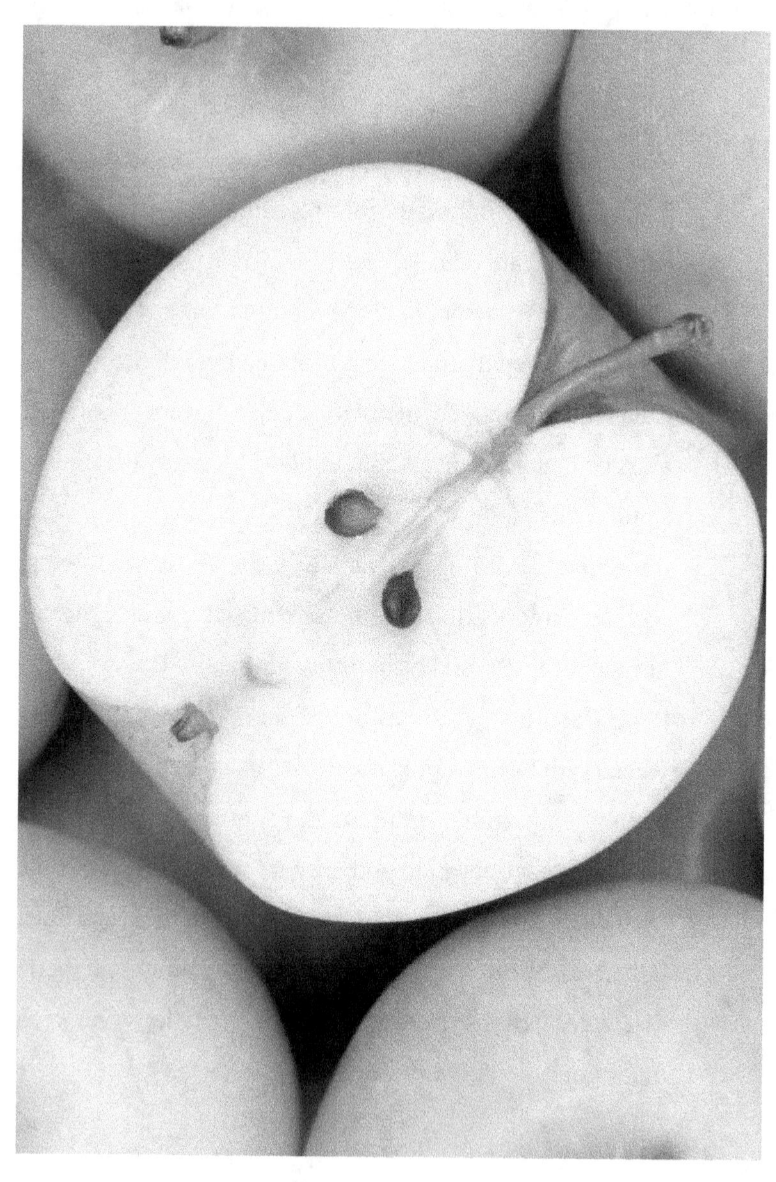

CHAPTER 2: 30-DAY MEAL PLAN

DAY 1

BREAKFAST: Avocado and Spinach Omelet

LUNCH: Lentil and Vegetable Stir-Fry

SNACK: Baked Kale Chips

DINNER: Lemon Herb Baked Chicken

DAY 2

BREAKFAST: Sweet Potato Breakfast Hash

LUNCH: Chickpea and Avocado Salad

SNACK: Avocado and Tomato Rice Cakes

DINNER: Vegetarian Lentil and Sweet Potato Curry

DAY 3

BREAKFAST: Greek Yogurt Parfait

LUNCH: Salmon and Quinoa Bowl with Lemon-Dill Dressing

SNACK: Cucumber and Hummus Bites

DINNER: Zucchini Noodles with Pesto and Cherry Tomatoes

DAY 4

BREAKFAST: Egg and Veggie Breakfast Muffins

LUNCH: Turkey and Vegetable Lettuce Wraps

SNACK: Egg and Avocado Rice Cake Stack

DINNER: Baked Lemon Garlic Herb Chicken Thighs

DAY 5

BREAKFAST: Almond Butter Banana Toast

LUNCH: Mediterranean Chickpea Salad

SNACK: Nut Butter Energy Balls

DINNER: Eggplant and Chickpea Curry

DAY 6

BREAKFAST: Millet Breakfast Porridge

LUNCH: Sesame Ginger Tofu Stir-Fry

SNACK: Apple and Almond Butter Slices

DINNER: Lemon Herb Baked Cod

DAY 7

BREAKFAST: Green Smoothie Bowl

LUNCH: Quinoa and Vegetable Stuffed Bell Peppers

SNACK: Carrot and Hummus Roll-Ups

DINNER: Chickpea and Vegetable Curry

DAY 8

BREAKFAST: Coconut Chia Pudding

LUNCH: Turkey and Vegetable Skillet with Quinoa

SNACK: Avocado and Tomato Rice Cakes

DINNER: Mediterranean Quinoa Salad with Grilled Chicken

DAY 9

BREAKFAST: Turmeric Scrambled Eggs with Sautéed Greens

LUNCH: Salmon and Asparagus Foil Packets

SNACK: Tuna and Avocado Cucumber Bites

DINNER: Salmon and Vegetable Foil Packets

DAY 10

BREAKFAST: Quinoa and Berry Breakfast Bowl

LUNCH: Turkey and Sweet Potato Hash

SNACK: Stuffed Bell Pepper Rings

DINNER: Stir-Fried Tofu with Broccoli and Cashews

DAY 11

BREAKFAST: Mushroom and Spinach Breakfast Wrap

LUNCH: Greek Chicken Salad Wrap

SNACK: Cucumber and Smoked Salmon Roll-Ups

DINNER: Lemon Garlic Shrimp with Quinoa

DAY 12

BREAKFAST: Buckwheat Pancakes with Mixed Berry Compote

LUNCH: Quinoa and Kale Stuffed Bell Peppers

SNACK: Sweet Potato and Almond Butter Bites

DINNER: Grilled Turkey and Vegetable Skewers

DAY 13

BREAKFAST: Chia Seed Pudding with Citrus Infusion

LUNCH: Mushroom and Spinach Quiche

SNACK: Cherry Tomato and Goat Cheese Stuffed Celery Sticks

DINNER: Vegetarian Lentil and Spinach Stuffed Bell Peppers

DAY 14

BREAKFAST: Mango-Coconut Overnight Oats

LUNCH: Vegetarian Quinoa and Black Bean Bowl

SNACK: Pomegranate and Cottage Cheese Parfait

DINNER: Turkey Stir-Fry with Bok Choy and Brown Rice Noodles

DAY 15

BREAKFAST: Lentil and Vegetable Breakfast Skillet

LUNCH: Caprese Chickpea Salad

SNACK: Tuna and Avocado Cucumber Bites

DINNER: Eggplant Lasagna with Ground Turkey and Tomato-Based Sauce

DAY 16

BREAKFAST: Avocado and Spinach Omelet

LUNCH: Lentil and Vegetable Stir-Fry

SNACK: Baked Kale Chips

DINNER: Lemon Herb Baked Chicken

DAY 17

BREAKFAST: Sweet Potato Breakfast Hash

LUNCH: Chickpea and Avocado Salad

SNACK: Avocado and Tomato Rice Cakes

DINNER: Vegetarian Lentil and Sweet Potato Curry

DAY 18

BREAKFAST: Greek Yogurt Parfait

LUNCH: Salmon and Quinoa Bowl with Lemon-Dill Dressing

SNACK: Cucumber and Hummus Bites

DINNER: Zucchini Noodles with Pesto and Cherry Tomatoes

DAY 19

BREAKFAST: Egg and Veggie Breakfast Muffins

LUNCH: Turkey and Vegetable Lettuce Wraps

SNACK: Egg and Avocado Rice Cake Stack

DINNER: Baked Lemon Garlic Herb Chicken Thighs

DAY 20

BREAKFAST: Almond Butter Banana Toast

LUNCH: Mediterranean Chickpea Salad

SNACK: Nut Butter Energy Balls

DINNER: Eggplant and Chickpea Curry

DAY 21

BREAKFAST: Millet Breakfast Porridge

LUNCH: Sesame Ginger Tofu Stir-Fry

SNACK: Apple and Almond Butter Slices

DINNER: Lemon Herb Baked Cod

DAY 22

BREAKFAST: Green Smoothie Bowl

LUNCH: Quinoa and Vegetable Stuffed Bell Peppers

SNACK: Carrot and Hummus Roll-Ups

DINNER: Chickpea and Vegetable Curry

DAY 23

BREAKFAST: Coconut Chia Pudding

LUNCH: Turkey and Vegetable Skillet with Quinoa

SNACK: Avocado and Tomato Rice Cakes

DINNER: Mediterranean Quinoa Salad with Grilled Chicken

DAY 24

BREAKFAST: Turmeric Scrambled Eggs with Sautéed Greens

LUNCH: Salmon and Asparagus Foil Packets

SNACK: Tuna and Avocado Cucumber Bites

DINNER: Salmon and Vegetable Foil Packets

DAY 25

BREAKFAST: Quinoa and Berry Breakfast Bowl

LUNCH: Turkey and Sweet Potato Hash

SNACK: Stuffed Bell Pepper Rings

DINNER: Stir-Fried Tofu with Broccoli and Cashews

DAY 26

BREAKFAST: Mushroom and Spinach Breakfast Wrap

LUNCH: Greek Chicken Salad Wrap

SNACK: Cucumber and Smoked Salmon Roll-Ups

DINNER: Lemon Garlic Shrimp with Quinoa

DAY 27

BREAKFAST: Buckwheat Pancakes with Mixed Berry Compote

LUNCH: Quinoa and Kale Stuffed Bell Peppers

SNACK: Sweet Potato and Almond Butter Bites

DINNER: Grilled Turkey and Vegetable Skewers

DAY 28

BREAKFAST: Chia Seed Pudding with Citrus Infusion

LUNCH: Mushroom and Spinach Quiche

SNACK: Cherry Tomato and Goat Cheese Stuffed Celery Sticks

DINNER: Vegetarian Lentil and Spinach Stuffed Bell Peppers

DAY 29

BREAKFAST: Mango-Coconut Overnight Oats

LUNCH: Vegetarian Quinoa and Black Bean Bowl

SNACK: Pomegranate and Cottage Cheese Parfait

DINNER: Turkey Stir-Fry with Bok Choy and Brown Rice Noodles

DAY 30

BREAKFAST: Lentil and Vegetable Breakfast Skillet

LUNCH: Caprese Chickpea Salad

SNACK: Tuna and Avocado Cucumber Bites

DINNER: Eggplant Lasagna with Ground Turkey and Tomato-Based Sauce

CHAPTER 3: BREAKFAST

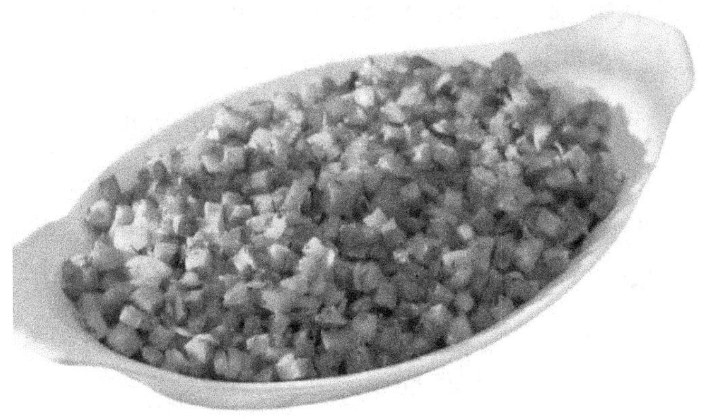

Avocado and Spinach Omelet

Ingredients:

- 2 eggs (organic, free-range)
- 1/2 avocado, sliced
- Handful of fresh spinach leaves
- 1/4 cup diced tomatoes
- 1/4 cup diced red bell pepper
- 1 tablespoon olive oil
- Salt and pepper to taste

Directions:

1. In a bowl, whisk the eggs until well beaten. Add a pinch of salt and pepper to taste.
2. Heat olive oil in a non-stick skillet over medium heat.

3. Add diced tomatoes and red bell pepper to the skillet, sauté for 2-3 minutes until slightly softened.

4. Add fresh spinach leaves to the skillet and cook until wilted.

5. Pour the beaten eggs over the vegetables in the skillet, swirling to ensure an even distribution.

6. Allow the eggs to set at the edges, then gently lift the edges with a spatula to let the uncooked eggs flow underneath.

7. Once the omelet is mostly set but still slightly runny on top, place avocado slices on one half of the omelet.

8. Carefully fold the other half of the omelet over the avocado, creating a half-moon shape.

9. Cook for an additional 1-2 minutes until the eggs are fully cooked but still moist inside.

10. Slide the omelet onto a plate and serve immediately.

Sweet Potato Breakfast Hash

Ingredients:

- 1 medium sweet potato, peeled and diced
- 1/2 cup diced red onion
- 1/2 cup diced bell peppers (any color)
- 1 cup baby spinach leaves
- 2 eggs (organic, free-range)

- 1 tablespoon olive oil
- Salt and pepper to taste
- Fresh herbs (such as parsley or chives) for garnish

Directions:

1. Heat olive oil in a skillet over medium heat.
2. Add diced sweet potatoes and sauté for 5-7 minutes until they start to soften.
3. Add diced red onion and bell peppers to the skillet, continue sautéing until vegetables are tender.
4. Stir in baby spinach leaves and cook until wilted.
5. Create two wells in the vegetable mixture and crack an egg into each well.
6. Cover the skillet and cook for 3-5 minutes until the eggs are cooked to your liking.
7. Season the hash with salt and pepper to taste.
8. Gently mix the eggs into the hash or leave them sunny-side-up, depending on your preference.
9. Sprinkle fresh herbs on top for added flavor.
10. Serve the sweet potato breakfast hash warm.

Greek Yogurt Parfait

Ingredients:

- 1 cup plain Greek yogurt

- 1/2 cup mixed berries (blueberries, raspberries, strawberries)
- 1/4 cup granola (look for a low-sugar option)
- 1 tablespoon raw honey
- 1 tablespoon chopped nuts (almonds, walnuts, or pistachios)
- 1/2 teaspoon vanilla extract (optional)

Directions:

1. In a glass or bowl, spoon a layer of Greek yogurt at the bottom.
2. Add a layer of mixed berries on top of the yogurt.
3. Sprinkle a portion of granola over the berries.
4. Drizzle raw honey over the granola for natural sweetness.
5. Repeat the layers until you've used all the ingredients or reached your desired serving size.
6. Top the parfait with a sprinkle of chopped nuts for added crunch.
7. If desired, add a splash of vanilla extract to the Greek yogurt for extra flavor.
8. Serve immediately and enjoy your nutritious Greek Yogurt Parfait!

Egg and Veggie Breakfast Muffins

Ingredients:

- 4 eggs (organic, free-range)
- 1/2 cup diced zucchini
- 1/2 cup diced cherry tomatoes
- 1/4 cup diced red onion
- 1/4 cup chopped spinach
- 1/4 cup feta cheese, crumbled
- 1 tablespoon olive oil
- Salt and pepper to taste
- Fresh herbs (such as parsley or chives) for garnish

Directions:

1. Preheat the oven to 350°F (175°C) and grease a muffin tin.
2. In a skillet, heat olive oil over medium heat.
3. Add diced zucchini, cherry tomatoes, and red onion to the skillet. Sauté until vegetables are tender.
4. Stir in chopped spinach and cook until wilted. Remove from heat.
5. In a bowl, beat the eggs and season with salt and pepper.
6. Add the sautéed vegetables and crumbled feta cheese to the beaten eggs. Mix well.
7. Spoon the mixture evenly into the muffin tin.

8. Bake in the preheated oven for 15-20 minutes or until the muffins are set and lightly golden.

9. Remove from the oven and let them cool for a few minutes.

10. Garnish with fresh herbs and serve these delicious egg and veggie breakfast muffins warm.

Almond Butter Banana Toast

Ingredients:

- 2 slices of sprouted grain or whole grain bread
- 2 tablespoons almond butter
- 1 ripe banana, sliced
- 1 teaspoon chia seeds
- 1 teaspoon honey (optional)
- Pinch of cinnamon for sprinkling

Directions:

1. Toast the slices of bread to your desired level of crispiness.

2. Spread a tablespoon of almond butter on each slice of toast.

3. Arrange sliced bananas on top of the almond butter.

4. Sprinkle chia seeds over the banana slices for added crunch and nutrition.

5. If desired, drizzle honey over the toast for sweetness.

6. Finish by lightly sprinkling cinnamon on top for flavor.

7. Serve the almond butter banana toast immediately.

Millet Breakfast Porridge

Ingredients:

- 1/2 cup millet, rinsed
- 1 cup almond milk (unsweetened)
- 1/2 cup diced apples
- 1 tablespoon chopped almonds
- 1/2 teaspoon ground cinnamon
- 1 teaspoon maple syrup (optional)
- Fresh berries for garnish

Directions:

1. In a saucepan, combine rinsed millet and almond milk. Bring to a boil.

2. Reduce heat to low, cover, and simmer for 15-20 minutes or until millet is tender and has absorbed most of the liquid.

3. Stir in diced apples, chopped almonds, and ground cinnamon. Cook for an additional 5 minutes.

4. If desired, sweeten the porridge with maple syrup, adjusting to your taste.

5. Remove from heat and let it sit, covered, for a few minutes to thicken.

6. Spoon the millet porridge into bowls and garnish with fresh berries.

7. Serve warm and enjoy this nutritious and hearty breakfast porridge.

Green Smoothie Bowl

Ingredients:

- 1 cup spinach leaves, packed
- 1/2 cup frozen mango chunks
- 1/2 ripe avocado
- 1/2 cup unsweetened almond milk
- 1 tablespoon chia seeds
- 1 tablespoon hemp seeds
- Sliced kiwi, banana, and berries for topping
- Granola for crunch (optional)

Directions:

1. In a blender, combine spinach, frozen mango, ripe avocado, almond milk, chia seeds, and hemp seeds.

2. Blend until smooth and creamy, adding more almond milk if needed for consistency.

3. Pour the green smoothie into a bowl.

4. Top the smoothie with sliced kiwi, banana, berries, and granola if desired.

5. Feel free to drizzle a bit of honey or maple syrup for added sweetness (optional).

6. Enjoy this nutrient-packed and refreshing green smoothie bowl.

Coconut Chia Pudding

Ingredients:

- 1/4 cup chia seeds
- 1 cup coconut milk (unsweetened)
- 1/2 teaspoon vanilla extract
- 1 tablespoon shredded coconut (unsweetened)
- 1/4 cup sliced strawberries
- 1/4 cup diced pineapple
- Mint leaves for garnish (optional)

Directions:

1. In a bowl, combine chia seeds, coconut milk, and vanilla extract. Stir well.

2. Let the mixture sit for 10 minutes, stirring occasionally to prevent clumping.

3. Once the chia seeds have absorbed the liquid and the mixture thickens, refrigerate for at least 2 hours or overnight.

4. Before serving, stir the chia pudding to ensure a smooth consistency.

5. In serving glasses or bowls, layer the chia pudding with shredded coconut.

6. Top with sliced strawberries, diced pineapple, and garnish with mint leaves if desired.

7. Serve chilled and enjoy this delightful coconut chia pudding for breakfast.

Turmeric Scrambled Eggs with Sautéed Greens

Ingredients:

- 2 eggs (organic, free-range)
- 1/2 teaspoon ground turmeric
- 1 tablespoon olive oil
- 1 cup mixed greens (spinach, kale, or Swiss chard), chopped
- 1/4 cup cherry tomatoes, halved
- 1 clove garlic, minced
- Salt and pepper to taste
- Fresh herbs (such as cilantro or parsley) for garnish

Directions:

1. In a bowl, whisk together the eggs and ground turmeric until well combined.

2. Heat olive oil in a skillet over medium heat.

3. Add minced garlic and sauté for a minute until fragrant.

4. Add the chopped mixed greens to the skillet and cook until wilted.

5. Pour the turmeric-spiced eggs into the skillet with the sautéed greens.

6. Gently scramble the eggs and mix them with the greens until fully cooked.

7. Season with salt and pepper to taste.

8. Add halved cherry tomatoes to the scrambled eggs and cook for an additional minute.

9. Remove from heat and transfer the scrambled eggs and greens to a plate.

10. Garnish with fresh herbs and serve this vibrant and nutritious breakfast.

Quinoa and Berry Breakfast Bowl

Ingredients:
- 1/2 cup cooked quinoa
- 1/2 cup mixed berries (blueberries, raspberries, strawberries)
- 1 tablespoon almond butter
- 1 tablespoon unsweetened shredded coconut
- 1 teaspoon chia seeds
- 1/2 teaspoon cinnamon
- 1/2 cup almond milk (unsweetened)

Directions:

1. In a bowl, combine cooked quinoa and mixed berries.

2. Drizzle almond butter over the quinoa and berries.

3. Sprinkle shredded coconut, chia seeds, and cinnamon on top.

4. Pour almond milk over the ingredients.

5. Gently mix everything together for an even distribution of flavors.

6. Allow the bowl to sit for a few minutes to let the chia seeds absorb some liquid.

7. Adjust sweetness with a touch of honey or maple syrup if desired.

8. Enjoy your nutritious and delicious quinoa and berry breakfast bowl!

Mushroom and Spinach Breakfast Wrap

Ingredients:

- 2 whole-grain or sprouted grain tortillas
- 1 cup sliced mushrooms
- 1 cup fresh spinach leaves
- 2 eggs (organic, free-range)
- 1 tablespoon olive oil
- 2 tablespoons feta cheese, crumbled
- Salt and pepper to taste

- Hot sauce or salsa for serving (optional)

Directions:

1. In a skillet, heat olive oil over medium heat.

2. Add sliced mushrooms to the skillet and sauté until they release their moisture and become golden brown.

3. Add fresh spinach leaves to the skillet and cook until wilted. Season with salt and pepper.

4. Push the mushrooms and spinach to one side of the skillet and crack the eggs into the other side.

5. Scramble the eggs until cooked through, then mix them with the mushrooms and spinach.

6. Warm the tortillas in the skillet or microwave.

7. Divide the egg, mushroom, and spinach mixture between the tortillas.

8. Sprinkle crumbled feta cheese over each wrap.

9. If desired, add a dash of hot sauce or salsa for extra flavor.

10. Fold the wraps and serve these savory mushroom and spinach breakfast wraps warm.

Buckwheat Pancakes with Mixed Berry Compote

Ingredients:

For Buckwheat Pancakes:

- 1 cup buckwheat flour
- 1 tablespoon ground flaxseed
- 1 teaspoon baking powder
- 1/2 teaspoon cinnamon
- 1 cup almond milk (unsweetened)
- 1 tablespoon maple syrup
- 1 tablespoon coconut oil (melted)
- 1 teaspoon vanilla extract

For Mixed Berry Compote:

- 1 cup mixed berries (blueberries, raspberries, strawberries)
- 1 tablespoon chia seeds
- 1 tablespoon maple syrup

Directions:

For Buckwheat Pancakes:

1. In a bowl, whisk together buckwheat flour, ground flaxseed, baking powder, and cinnamon.
2. In a separate bowl, combine almond milk, maple syrup, melted coconut oil, and vanilla extract.

3. Pour the wet ingredients into the dry ingredients and stir until just combined.

4. Heat a griddle or non-stick pan over medium heat.

5. Pour 1/4 cup of batter for each pancake onto the griddle.

6. Cook until bubbles form on the surface, then flip and cook until both sides are golden brown.

7. Repeat with the remaining batter.

For Mixed Berry Compote:

1. In a small saucepan, combine mixed berries, chia seeds, and maple syrup.

2. Cook over medium heat until the berries break down and the mixture thickens, stirring occasionally.

3. Remove from heat and let it cool for a few minutes.

Assembly:

1. Stack the buckwheat pancakes on a plate.

2. Spoon the mixed berry compote over the pancakes.

3. Optionally, drizzle with additional maple syrup.

4. Serve warm and enjoy this delightful and nutritious breakfast!

Chia Seed Pudding with Citrus Infusion

Ingredients:

- 1/4 cup chia seeds
- 1 cup coconut milk (unsweetened)

- Zest of 1 orange
- Zest of 1 lemon
- 1 tablespoon maple syrup or honey (optional)
- Sliced citrus fruits (orange, grapefruit, or a mix)
- Fresh mint leaves for garnish

Directions:

1. In a bowl, whisk together chia seeds, coconut milk, citrus zests, and maple syrup or honey if using.
2. Allow the mixture to sit for a few minutes, then whisk again to prevent clumps.
3. Refrigerate the chia seed mixture for at least 2 hours or overnight until it thickens.
4. Stir the pudding before serving to ensure a smooth consistency.
5. Spoon the chia seed pudding into serving glasses or bowls.
6. Top with slices of citrus fruits for a burst of freshness.
7. Garnish with fresh mint leaves.
8. Serve chilled and enjoy this refreshing chia seed pudding with citrus infusion for breakfast.

Mango-Coconut Overnight Oats

Ingredients:

- 1/2 cup rolled oats

- 1/2 cup coconut milk (unsweetened)
- 1/4 cup diced mango
- 1 tablespoon chia seeds
- 1 tablespoon shredded coconut (unsweetened)
- 1 teaspoon honey or maple syrup (optional)
- Sliced almonds for topping
- Fresh mint leaves for garnish (optional)

Directions:

1. In a jar or bowl, combine rolled oats, coconut milk, diced mango, chia seeds, and shredded coconut.
2. If desired, sweeten with honey or maple syrup, adjusting to your taste.
3. Stir well to ensure all ingredients are evenly mixed.
4. Cover the jar or bowl and refrigerate overnight or for at least 4 hours to allow the oats and chia seeds to absorb the liquid.
5. Before serving, give the mixture a good stir to achieve a creamy consistency.
6. Top the overnight oats with sliced almonds for added crunch.
7. Garnish with fresh mint leaves if desired.
8. Enjoy this tropical-inspired mango-coconut overnight oats for a quick and nutritious breakfast!

Lentil and Vegetable Breakfast Skillet

Ingredients:

- 1/2 cup cooked green lentils
- 1/2 cup diced zucchini
- 1/2 cup cherry tomatoes, halved
- 1/4 cup diced red onion
- 2 eggs (organic, free-range)
- 1 tablespoon olive oil
- 1 teaspoon ground cumin
- 1/2 teaspoon smoked paprika
- Salt and pepper to taste
- Fresh cilantro for garnish (optional)

Directions:

1. In a skillet, heat olive oil over medium heat.
2. Add diced zucchini, cherry tomatoes, and red onion to the skillet. Sauté until vegetables are tender.
3. Stir in cooked green lentils, ground cumin, smoked paprika, salt, and pepper. Cook for an additional 2-3 minutes.
4. Create two wells in the lentil and vegetable mixture and crack an egg into each well.
5. Cover the skillet and cook for 3-5 minutes until the eggs are cooked to your liking.

6. If desired, sprinkle fresh cilantro on top for added freshness.

7. Serve this lentil and vegetable breakfast skillet warm.

Tofu Scramble with Spinach and Tomatoes

Ingredients:

- 1/2 block firm tofu, crumbled
- 1 cup fresh spinach leaves, chopped
- 1/2 cup cherry tomatoes, halved
- 1/4 cup diced red bell pepper
- 2 tablespoons nutritional yeast
- 1 tablespoon olive oil
- 1 teaspoon turmeric powder
- 1/2 teaspoon garlic powder
- Salt and pepper to taste
- Fresh parsley for garnish (optional)

Directions:

1. In a skillet, heat olive oil over medium heat.

2. Add crumbled tofu to the skillet and cook for 2-3 minutes.

3. Stir in turmeric powder, garlic powder, salt, and pepper. Mix well to coat the tofu.

4. Add chopped spinach, cherry tomatoes, and diced red bell pepper to the skillet. Sauté until the vegetables are tender.

5. Sprinkle nutritional yeast over the mixture and stir to incorporate.

6. Cook for an additional 2-3 minutes, allowing the flavors to meld.

7. Taste and adjust seasoning if needed.

8. Garnish with fresh parsley if desired.

9. Serve this tofu scramble with spinach and tomatoes warm.

Buckwheat Banana Pancakes

Ingredients:

- 1/2 cup buckwheat flour
- 1 ripe banana, mashed
- 1/2 cup almond milk (unsweetened)
- 1 egg (organic, free-range)
- 1 teaspoon baking powder
- 1/2 teaspoon cinnamon
- 1/4 teaspoon vanilla extract
- Pinch of salt
- Coconut oil for cooking

Directions:

1. In a mixing bowl, combine buckwheat flour, mashed banana, almond milk, egg, baking powder, cinnamon, vanilla extract, and a pinch of salt. Mix until well combined.
2. Heat a skillet or griddle over medium heat and add a small amount of coconut oil.
3. Pour 1/4 cup portions of batter onto the skillet to form pancakes.
4. Cook until bubbles form on the surface, then flip and cook the other side until golden brown.
5. Repeat until all the batter is used, adding more coconut oil as needed.
6. Serve the buckwheat banana pancakes warm.

Millet Breakfast Bowl with Almond Butter and Berries

Ingredients:

- 1/2 cup cooked millet
- 2 tablespoons almond butter
- 1/2 cup mixed berries (blueberries, strawberries, raspberries)
- 1 tablespoon chia seeds
- 1 tablespoon unsweetened shredded coconut

- 1 teaspoon honey (optional)

Directions:

1. In a bowl, combine cooked millet and almond butter, stirring until well mixed.

2. Add mixed berries on top of the millet-almond butter mixture.

3. Sprinkle chia seeds and shredded coconut over the berries.

4. If desired, drizzle honey over the bowl for added sweetness.

5. Gently mix all ingredients to ensure an even distribution of flavors.

6. Allow the bowl to sit for a few minutes to let the chia seeds absorb some liquid.

7. Adjust sweetness and toppings according to your preferences.

8. Enjoy your nutritious and delicious millet breakfast bowl with almond butter and berries!

Avocado and Smoked Salmon Rice Cakes

Ingredients:

- 2 rice cakes (choose whole grain or brown rice)
- 1/2 ripe avocado, sliced
- 2 oz smoked salmon

- 1 tablespoon lemon juice
- 1 tablespoon capers
- Fresh dill for garnish
- Black pepper to taste

Directions:

1. Place the rice cakes on a serving plate.

2. Arrange avocado slices on top of each rice cake.

3. Drape smoked salmon over the avocado.

4. Drizzle lemon juice over the avocado and salmon.

5. Sprinkle capers evenly on the rice cakes.

6. Finish with a pinch of black pepper for added flavor.

7. Garnish with fresh dill leaves.

8. Serve these avocado and smoked salmon rice cakes immediately.

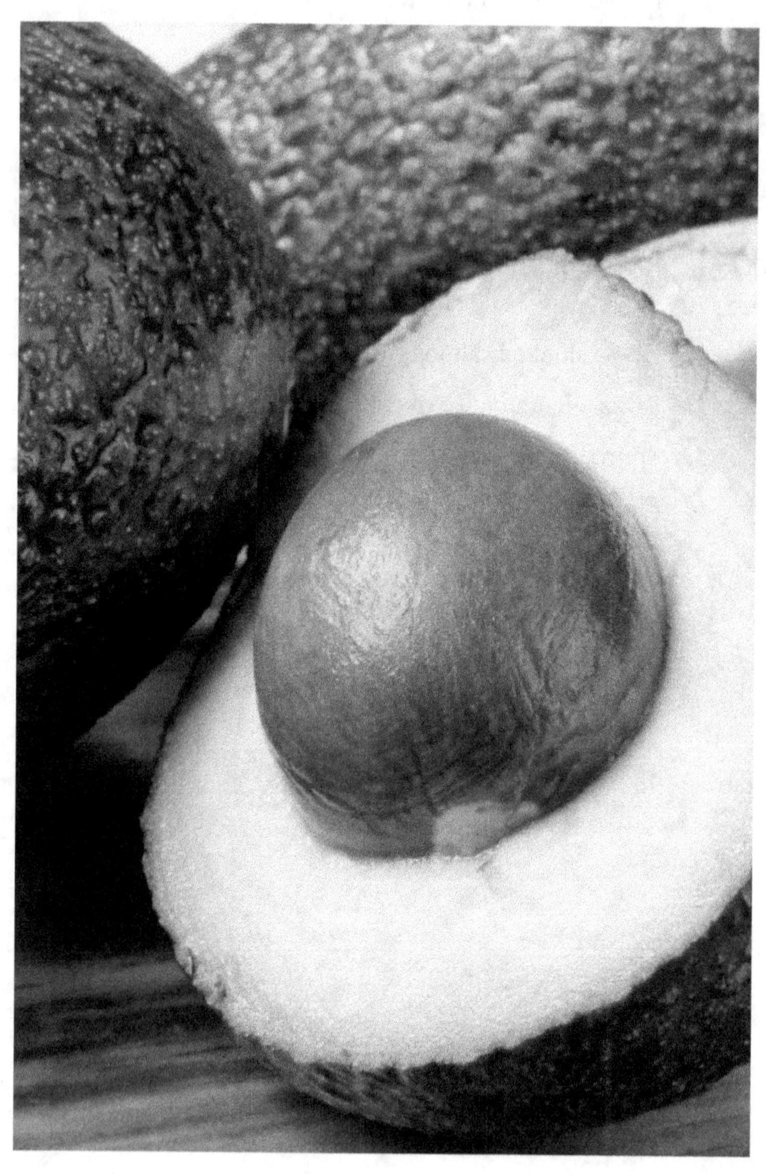

CHAPTER 4: LUNCH

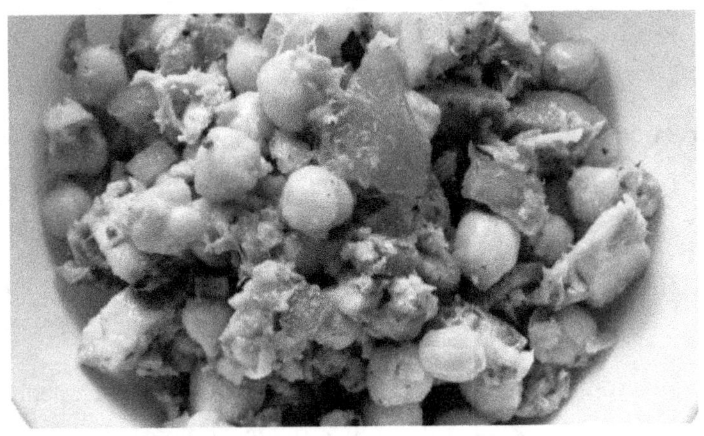

Lentil and Vegetable Stir-Fry

Ingredients:

- 1 cup cooked green lentils
- 1 cup broccoli florets
- 1 medium carrot, julienned
- 1/2 red bell pepper, sliced
- 1/2 yellow bell pepper, sliced
- 1/2 cup snap peas, ends trimmed
- 2 cloves garlic, minced
- 1 tablespoon ginger, grated
- 2 tablespoons tamari or soy sauce (low-sodium)
- 1 tablespoon sesame oil
- 1 tablespoon olive oil

- 1 tablespoon rice vinegar
- 1 teaspoon honey or maple syrup (optional)
- Sesame seeds for garnish
- Green onions, chopped, for garnish

Directions:

1. In a large skillet or wok, heat olive oil over medium-high heat.
2. Add minced garlic and grated ginger to the skillet, sautéing for 1-2 minutes until fragrant.
3. Add broccoli, carrot, red bell pepper, yellow bell pepper, and snap peas to the skillet. Stir-fry for 5-7 minutes until vegetables are tender-crisp.
4. Stir in the cooked green lentils, mixing well with the vegetables.
5. In a small bowl, whisk together tamari or soy sauce, sesame oil, rice vinegar, and honey or maple syrup if using.
6. Pour the sauce over the lentil and vegetable mixture. Stir to coat evenly.
7. Continue to cook for an additional 2-3 minutes until everything is heated through.
8. Taste and adjust the seasoning if needed.
9. Garnish the stir-fry with sesame seeds and chopped green onions.

10. Serve this lentil and vegetable stir-fry over brown rice or quinoa for a wholesome and satisfying lunch.

Chickpea and Avocado Salad

Ingredients:

- 1 can (15 oz) chickpeas, drained and rinsed
- 1 ripe avocado, diced
- 1 cup cherry tomatoes, halved
- 1/4 cup red onion, finely chopped
- 1/4 cup cucumber, diced
- 2 tablespoons fresh parsley, chopped
- 1 tablespoon olive oil
- 1 tablespoon lemon juice
- 1 teaspoon Dijon mustard
- Salt and pepper to taste
- Mixed salad greens for serving

Directions:

1. In a large bowl, combine chickpeas, diced avocado, cherry tomatoes, red onion, cucumber, and fresh parsley.
2. In a small bowl, whisk together olive oil, lemon juice, Dijon mustard, salt, and pepper to create the dressing.
3. Pour the dressing over the chickpea and avocado mixture. Gently toss to coat everything evenly.

4. Let the salad marinate for a few minutes to enhance the flavors.

5. Arrange a bed of mixed salad greens on a plate.

6. Spoon the chickpea and avocado salad over the greens.

7. Optional: Garnish with additional parsley for freshness.

8. Serve this refreshing chickpea and avocado salad as a light and satisfying lunch.

Salmon and Quinoa Bowl with Lemon-Dill Dressing

Ingredients:

- 1 cup cooked quinoa
- 6 oz salmon filet
- 1 tablespoon olive oil
- 1/2 teaspoon garlic powder
- Salt and pepper to taste
- 1 cup mixed greens (spinach, arugula, or your choice)
- 1/2 cucumber, sliced
- 1/4 cup cherry tomatoes, halved
- 1/4 cup red bell pepper, diced
- 1 tablespoon fresh dill, chopped

Lemon-Dill Dressing:

- 2 tablespoons olive oil
- 1 tablespoon lemon juice

- 1 teaspoon Dijon mustard
- 1 teaspoon honey or maple syrup (optional)
- Salt and pepper to taste

Directions:

1. Preheat the oven to 400°F (200°C).
2. Place the salmon filet on a baking sheet, drizzle with olive oil, and sprinkle with garlic powder, salt, and pepper.
3. Bake the salmon for 12-15 minutes or until it flakes easily with a fork.
4. In a bowl, combine cooked quinoa, mixed greens, cucumber slices, cherry tomatoes, and diced red bell pepper.
5. Flake the baked salmon and add it to the quinoa bowl.
6. In a small bowl, whisk together olive oil, lemon juice, Dijon mustard, honey or maple syrup, salt and pepper to create the dressing.
7. Drizzle the lemon-dill dressing over the quinoa bowl and toss gently to coat.
8. Sprinkle fresh chopped dill on top for added flavor.
9. Serve this salmon and quinoa bowl for a delicious and nutritious lunch.

Turkey and Vegetable Lettuce Wraps

Ingredients:

- 1/2 lb ground turkey
- 1 tablespoon olive oil
- 1/2 cup bell peppers, diced (mix of colors)
- 1/4 cup shredded carrots
- 2 green onions, sliced
- 1 clove garlic, minced
- 1 teaspoon ginger, grated
- 2 tablespoons tamari or soy sauce (low-sodium)
- 1 tablespoon hoisin sauce
- Butter lettuce leaves for wrapping

Optional Toppings:

- Sesame seeds
- Chopped cilantro
- Sliced radishes

Directions:

1. In a skillet, heat olive oil over medium-high heat.
2. Add ground turkey to the skillet and cook until browned, breaking it apart with a spoon as it cooks.
3. Add diced bell peppers, shredded carrots, green onions, minced garlic, and grated ginger to the skillet. Sauté for 3-4 minutes until vegetables are tender.

4. In a small bowl, mix tamari or soy sauce and hoisin sauce. Pour the sauce over the turkey and vegetable mixture. Stir to combine and cook for an additional 2-3 minutes.

5. Remove from heat and let it cool slightly.

6. Spoon the turkey and vegetable mixture into butter lettuce leaves, creating wraps.

7. Optional: Top with sesame seeds, chopped cilantro, and sliced radishes for extra flavor and crunch.

8. Serve these turkey and vegetable lettuce wraps as a light and satisfying lunch.

Mediterranean Chickpea Salad

Ingredients:

- 1 can (15 oz) chickpeas, drained and rinsed
- 1 cup cherry tomatoes, halved
- 1 cucumber, diced
- 1/4 cup red onion, finely chopped
- 1/4 cup Kalamata olives, sliced
- 1/4 cup feta cheese, crumbled
- 2 tablespoons extra-virgin olive oil
- 1 tablespoon balsamic vinegar
- 1 teaspoon dried oregano
- Salt and pepper to taste

- Fresh parsley for garnish (optional)

Directions:

1. In a large bowl, combine chickpeas, cherry tomatoes, diced cucumber, red onion, Kalamata olives, and crumbled feta cheese.
2. In a small bowl, whisk together extra-virgin olive oil, balsamic vinegar, dried oregano, salt, and pepper to create the dressing.
3. Pour the dressing over the chickpea mixture. Gently toss to coat all ingredients evenly.
4. Let the salad marinate for a few minutes to enhance the flavors.
5. Optional: Garnish with fresh parsley for added freshness.
6. Serve this Mediterranean chickpea salad as a light and nutritious lunch.

Sesame Ginger Tofu Stir-Fry

Ingredients:

- 1 block firm tofu, cubed
- 2 tablespoons sesame oil
- 2 tablespoons tamari or soy sauce (low-sodium)
- 1 tablespoon rice vinegar
- 1 tablespoon honey or maple syrup
- 1 tablespoon fresh ginger, grated

- 2 cloves garlic, minced
- 1 cup broccoli florets
- 1/2 cup snap peas, trimmed
- 1 carrot, julienned
- 1 bell pepper, thinly sliced
- 2 green onions, sliced
- 1 tablespoon sesame seeds for garnish
- Cooked brown rice for serving

Directions:

1. In a bowl, whisk together sesame oil, tamari or soy sauce, rice vinegar, honey or maple syrup, grated ginger, and minced garlic to create the sauce.

2. Press excess water from the tofu by placing it between paper towels and gently pressing. Cube the tofu.

3. Heat a large skillet or wok over medium-high heat. Add cubed tofu and stir-fry until golden brown on all sides.

4. Remove tofu from the skillet and set aside.

5. In the same skillet, add a bit more sesame oil if needed. Add broccoli, snap peas, julienned carrot, and sliced bell pepper. Stir-fry for 3-4 minutes until vegetables are tender-crisp.

6. Add the cooked tofu back to the skillet and pour the sauce over the tofu and vegetables. Stir to coat everything evenly and cook for an additional 2-3 minutes.

7. Stir in sliced green onions.

8. Optional: Sprinkle sesame seeds over the stir-fry for added crunch.

9. Serve this sesame ginger tofu stir-fry over cooked brown rice for a delicious and satisfying lunch.

Quinoa and Vegetable Stuffed Bell Peppers

Ingredients:

- 4 large bell peppers, halved and seeds removed
- 1 cup cooked quinoa
- 1 can (15 oz) black beans, drained and rinsed
- 1 cup corn kernels (fresh or frozen)
- 1 cup cherry tomatoes, halved
- 1/2 cup red onion, finely chopped
- 1/2 cup cilantro, chopped
- 1 teaspoon ground cumin
- 1 teaspoon chili powder
- Salt and pepper to taste
- 1 cup shredded cheese (cheddar or your choice)
- Salsa for serving (optional)

- Avocado slices for garnish (optional)

Directions:

1. Preheat the oven to 375°F (190°C).

2. In a large mixing bowl, combine cooked quinoa, black beans, corn, cherry tomatoes, red onion, cilantro, ground cumin, chili powder, salt, and pepper. Mix well.

3. Place the halved bell peppers in a baking dish.

4. Spoon the quinoa and vegetable mixture into each bell pepper half, pressing it down slightly.

5. Top each stuffed pepper with shredded cheese.

6. Cover the baking dish with foil and bake in the preheated oven for 25-30 minutes or until the peppers are tender.

7. Remove the foil and broil for an additional 2-3 minutes until the cheese is bubbly and golden.

8. Optional: Serve the stuffed bell peppers with salsa and garnish with avocado slices.

9. Enjoy these quinoa and vegetable stuffed bell peppers as a wholesome and easy-to-make lunch.

Eggplant and Chickpea Buddha Bowl

Ingredients:

- 1 medium eggplant, sliced
- 1 can (15 oz) chickpeas, drained and rinsed

- 2 tablespoons olive oil

- 1 teaspoon ground cumin

- 1 teaspoon smoked paprika

- Salt and pepper to taste

- 2 cups cooked quinoa

- 1 cup cherry tomatoes, halved

- 1/2 cucumber, diced

- 1/4 cup red onion, finely chopped

- 1/4 cup fresh parsley, chopped

- Juice of 1 lemon

- Tahini dressing (store-bought or homemade)

Directions:

1. Preheat the oven to 400°F (200°C).

2. Place eggplant slices on a baking sheet, drizzle with olive oil, and sprinkle with ground cumin, smoked paprika, salt, and pepper.

3. Roast the eggplant in the preheated oven for 20-25 minutes or until tender and golden.

4. In a separate bowl, toss chickpeas with a bit of olive oil, cumin, smoked paprika, salt, and pepper. Spread them on a baking sheet and roast for 15-20 minutes or until crispy.

5. In serving bowls, assemble the Buddha bowls with cooked quinoa, roasted eggplant, roasted chickpeas, cherry tomatoes, diced cucumber, red onion, and fresh parsley.

6. Drizzle lemon juice over the bowls for freshness.

7. Serve the Buddha bowls with tahini dressing on the side for drizzling.

Turkey and Vegetable Skillet with Quinoa

Ingredients:

- 1 cup quinoa, rinsed
- 1 lb ground turkey
- 1 tablespoon olive oil
- 1 onion, finely chopped
- 2 cloves garlic, minced
- 1 bell pepper, diced (any color)
- 1 zucchini, diced
- 1 cup cherry tomatoes, halved
- 1 teaspoon dried oregano
- 1 teaspoon ground cumin
- Salt and pepper to taste
- Fresh parsley for garnish

Directions:

1. In a medium saucepan, cook quinoa according to package instructions. Set aside.
2. In a large skillet, heat olive oil over medium-high heat.
3. Add chopped onion and minced garlic, sautéing until softened.
4. Add ground turkey to the skillet, breaking it apart with a spoon. Cook until browned.
5. Stir in diced bell pepper and zucchini. Cook for 3-4 minutes until vegetables are tender.
6. Add halved cherry tomatoes to the skillet and cook for an additional 2 minutes.
7. Season the mixture with dried oregano, ground cumin, salt, and pepper. Stir well to combine.
8. Combine the cooked quinoa with the turkey and vegetable mixture in the skillet. Mix until everything is evenly distributed.
9. Garnish with fresh parsley.
10. Serve this turkey and vegetable skillet over quinoa as a delicious and easy-to-make lunch.

Salmon and Asparagus Foil Packets

Ingredients:

- 2 salmon filets

- 1 bunch asparagus, trimmed
- 1 lemon, sliced
- 2 tablespoons olive oil
- 2 cloves garlic, minced
- 1 teaspoon dried dill
- Salt and pepper to taste
- Fresh parsley for garnish

Directions:

1. Preheat the oven to 400°F (200°C).
2. Cut two large pieces of aluminum foil.
3. Place a salmon filet on each piece of foil.
4. Arrange trimmed asparagus around the salmon filets.
5. In a small bowl, whisk together olive oil, minced garlic, dried dill, salt, and pepper.
6. Drizzle the olive oil mixture over the salmon and asparagus.
7. Place lemon slices on top of each salmon filet.
8. Fold and seal the foil packets, ensuring they are well-enclosed.
9. Bake in the preheated oven for 15-20 minutes or until the salmon is cooked through and flakes easily.
10. Carefully open the foil packets, garnish with fresh parsley, and serve.

Quinoa and Kale Stuffed Bell Peppers

Ingredients:

- 4 bell peppers, halved and seeds removed
- 1 cup quinoa, cooked
- 2 cups kale, chopped
- 1 can (15 oz) black beans, drained and rinsed
- 1 cup cherry tomatoes, diced
- 1/2 cup red onion, finely chopped
- 1 teaspoon ground cumin
- 1 teaspoon paprika
- Salt and pepper to taste
- 1 cup shredded Monterey Jack or your favorite cheese
- Fresh cilantro for garnish
- Lime wedges for serving

Directions:

1. Preheat the oven to 375°F (190°C).
2. Place the bell pepper halves in a baking dish.
3. In a large bowl, combine cooked quinoa, chopped kale, black beans, cherry tomatoes, red onion, ground cumin, paprika, salt, and pepper.
4. Spoon the quinoa mixture into each bell pepper half, pressing it down gently.
5. Sprinkle shredded cheese over the top of each stuffed pepper.

6. Cover the baking dish with foil and bake for 25-30 minutes or until the peppers are tender.

7. Remove the foil and broil for an additional 2-3 minutes until the cheese is melted and golden.

8. Garnish with fresh cilantro.

9. Serve these quinoa and kale stuffed bell peppers with lime wedges on the side.

Mushroom and Spinach Quiche

Ingredients:

- 1 whole-grain pie crust (store-bought or homemade)
- 1 cup mushrooms, sliced
- 2 cups fresh spinach, chopped
- 1/2 cup red onion, finely chopped
- 3 eggs
- 1 cup milk (dairy or plant-based)
- 1/2 cup feta cheese, crumbled
- 1 teaspoon olive oil
- Salt and pepper to taste
- Fresh thyme for garnish

Directions:

1. Preheat the oven to 375°F (190°C).

2. In a skillet, heat olive oil over medium heat. Add sliced mushrooms and chopped red onion.

3. Sauté until mushrooms release their moisture and onions are softened.

4. Add chopped spinach to the skillet and cook until wilted. Remove from heat and let it cool slightly.

5. In a bowl, whisk together eggs and milk. Season with salt and pepper.

6. Place the pie crust in a pie dish.

7. Spread the mushroom, spinach, and onion mixture evenly over the pie crust.

8. Pour the egg and milk mixture over the vegetables.

9. Sprinkle crumbled feta cheese on top.

10. Bake in the preheated oven for 30-35 minutes or until the quiche is set and the crust is golden brown.

11. Garnish with fresh thyme before serving.

Turkey and Sweet Potato Hash

Ingredients:

- 1 lb ground turkey
- 2 medium sweet potatoes, peeled and diced
- 1 red bell pepper, diced
- 1 yellow onion, finely chopped
- 2 cloves garlic, minced
- 1 teaspoon smoked paprika
- 1 teaspoon dried thyme

- Salt and pepper to taste

- 2 tablespoons olive oil

- Fresh parsley for garnish

Directions:

1. In a large skillet, heat olive oil over medium-high heat.

2. Add chopped onion and minced garlic, sautéing until softened.

3. Add ground turkey to the skillet, breaking it apart with a spoon. Cook until browned.

4. Add diced sweet potatoes and diced red bell pepper to the skillet. Stir well.

5. Season the mixture with smoked paprika, dried thyme, salt, and pepper. Mix to combine.

6. Cover the skillet and cook for 15-20 minutes, stirring occasionally, until sweet potatoes are tender.

7. If needed, add a splash of water to prevent sticking and ensure even cooking.

8. Once the sweet potatoes are cooked through, adjust the seasoning to taste.

9. Garnish the turkey and sweet potato hash with fresh parsley.

10. Serve this flavorful and hearty hash for a satisfying and easy-to-make lunch.

Greek Chicken Salad Wrap

Ingredients:

- 1 cup cooked chicken breast, shredded or diced
- 1 whole-grain or sprouted grain wrap
- 1/2 cup cherry tomatoes, halved
- 1/4 cup cucumber, diced
- 1/4 cup red onion, finely chopped
- 1/4 cup Kalamata olives, sliced
- 1/4 cup feta cheese, crumbled
- 2 tablespoons Greek yogurt
- 1 tablespoon extra-virgin olive oil
- 1 tablespoon lemon juice
- 1 teaspoon dried oregano
- Salt and pepper to taste
- Fresh parsley for garnish

Directions:

1. In a bowl, combine cooked chicken breast, cherry tomatoes, diced cucumber, chopped red onion, sliced Kalamata olives, and crumbled feta cheese.

2. In a separate small bowl, whisk together Greek yogurt, extra-virgin olive oil, lemon juice, dried oregano, salt, and pepper to create the dressing.

3. Pour the dressing over the chicken and vegetable mixture. Toss to coat everything evenly.

4. Warm the wrap slightly if desired.

5. Spoon the Greek chicken salad onto the center of the wrap.

6. Optional: Garnish with fresh parsley for added freshness.

7. Fold in the sides of the wrap and then roll it up tightly.

8. Slice the wrap in half at a diagonal.

9. Serve this Greek chicken salad wrap as a delicious and easy-to-make lunch.

Vegetarian Quinoa and Black Bean Bowl

Ingredients:

- 1 cup quinoa, cooked
- 1 can (15 oz) black beans, drained and rinsed
- 1 cup corn kernels (fresh or frozen)
- 1 avocado, diced
- 1 cup cherry tomatoes, halved
- 1/4 cup red onion, finely chopped
- 1/4 cup fresh cilantro, chopped
- Juice of 1 lime
- 2 tablespoons olive oil
- 1 teaspoon ground cumin
- Salt and pepper to taste

Directions:

1. In a large bowl, combine cooked quinoa, black beans, corn, diced avocado, cherry tomatoes, and chopped red onion.
2. In a small bowl, whisk together olive oil, lime juice, ground cumin, salt, and pepper to create the dressing.
3. Pour the dressing over the quinoa and black bean mixture. Toss gently to coat everything evenly.
4. Sprinkle fresh cilantro on top for added flavor.
5. Allow the bowl to sit for a few minutes to let the flavors meld.
6. Serve this vegetarian quinoa and black bean bowl as a refreshing and easy-to-make lunch.

Caprese Chickpea Salad

Ingredients:

- 1 can (15 oz) chickpeas, drained and rinsed
- 1 cup cherry tomatoes, halved
- 1 cup fresh mozzarella cheese, diced
- 1/4 cup fresh basil leaves, torn
- 1 tablespoon extra-virgin olive oil
- Balsamic glaze for drizzling
- Salt and pepper to taste

Directions:

1. In a large bowl, combine chickpeas, cherry tomatoes, diced fresh mozzarella, and torn basil leaves.
2. Drizzle extra-virgin olive oil over the salad.
3. Gently toss the ingredients to coat them evenly.
4. Season with salt and pepper to taste.
5. Drizzle balsamic glaze over the salad for added sweetness and depth of flavor.
6. Allow the salad to marinate for a few minutes to enhance the flavors.
7. Serve this Caprese chickpea salad as a light and easy-to-make lunch.

Miso-Glazed Salmon Salad

Ingredients:

- 2 salmon filets
- 4 cups mixed salad greens (e.g., spinach, arugula, and watercress)
- 1 cucumber, thinly sliced
- 1 carrot, julienned
- 1/4 cup radishes, thinly sliced
- 2 tablespoons miso paste
- 1 tablespoon honey
- 1 tablespoon soy sauce (low-sodium)

- 1 tablespoon rice vinegar
- 1 teaspoon grated ginger
- 1 clove garlic, minced
- 2 tablespoons sesame oil
- Sesame seeds for garnish
- Sliced green onions for garnish

Directions:

1. Preheat the oven to 400°F (200°C).
2. In a small bowl, mix miso paste, honey, soy sauce, rice vinegar, grated ginger, minced garlic, and sesame oil to create the glaze.
3. Place salmon filets on a baking sheet lined with parchment paper.
4. Brush the miso glaze over the salmon filets.
5. Bake in the preheated oven for 12-15 minutes or until the salmon is cooked through and flakes easily.
6. While the salmon is baking, assemble the salad by combining mixed greens, sliced cucumber, julienned carrot, and sliced radishes in a large bowl.
7. Once the salmon is done, let it cool for a few minutes, then flake it into bite-sized pieces.
8. Arrange the flaked salmon over the salad.
9. Drizzle any remaining miso glaze over the salad.
10. Garnish with sesame seeds and sliced green onions.

11. Serve this miso-glazed salmon salad as a flavorful and easy-to-make lunch.

Sweet Potato and Lentil Buddha Bowl

Ingredients:

- 1 cup cooked lentils
- 1 medium sweet potato, peeled and diced
- 1 cup broccoli florets
- 1 tablespoon olive oil
- 1 teaspoon ground turmeric
- 1 teaspoon ground cumin
- Salt and pepper to taste
- 2 cups cooked quinoa
- 1/2 avocado, sliced
- 1/4 cup pumpkin seeds
- Tahini dressing (store-bought or homemade)

Directions:

1. Preheat the oven to 400°F (200°C).
2. Toss diced sweet potato and broccoli florets with olive oil, ground turmeric, ground cumin, salt, and pepper.
3. Spread the sweet potato and broccoli on a baking sheet in a single layer.
4. Roast in the preheated oven for 20-25 minutes or until the sweet potato is tender and slightly crispy.

5. While the vegetables are roasting, assemble the Buddha bowls. Start with a base of cooked quinoa.

6. Top the quinoa with cooked lentils, roasted sweet potato, and broccoli.

7. Add sliced avocado on the side of the bowl.

8. Sprinkle pumpkin seeds over the bowl for crunch.

9. Drizzle with tahini dressing.

10. Serve this sweet potato and lentil Buddha bowl as a wholesome and easy-to-make lunch.

Spinach and Feta Stuffed Turkey Burgers

Ingredients:

- 1 lb ground turkey
- 2 cups fresh spinach, chopped
- 1/2 cup feta cheese, crumbled
- 1/4 cup red onion, finely chopped
- 1 clove garlic, minced
- 1 teaspoon dried oregano
- Salt and pepper to taste
- Whole-grain burger buns
- Toppings: Tomato slices, cucumber, lettuce

Directions:

1. In a large bowl, combine ground turkey, chopped spinach, crumbled feta, chopped red onion, minced garlic, dried oregano, salt, and pepper.
2. Mix the ingredients until well combined.
3. Divide the mixture into equal portions and shape them into burger patties.
4. Heat a grill or skillet over medium-high heat.
5. Cook the turkey burgers for 4-5 minutes per side or until they are cooked through and have a golden brown exterior.
6. Optional: Toast the whole-grain burger buns on the grill or in a toaster.
7. Assemble the burgers by placing the turkey patties on the buns.
8. Add your favorite toppings such as tomato slices, cucumber, and lettuce.
9. Serve these spinach and feta stuffed turkey burgers as a flavorful and easy-to-make lunch.

Turmeric Chicken and Vegetable Skewers

Ingredients:

- 1 lb boneless, skinless chicken breasts, cut into chunks
- 1 zucchini, sliced

- 1 bell pepper, diced
- 1 red onion, cut into chunks
- 1 tablespoon olive oil
- 1 teaspoon ground turmeric
- 1 teaspoon paprika
- 1 teaspoon cumin
- Salt and pepper to taste
- Wooden skewers, soaked in water

Directions:

1. Preheat the grill or grill pan over medium-high heat.
2. In a bowl, mix olive oil, ground turmeric, paprika, cumin, salt, and pepper to create a marinade.
3. Thread chicken chunks, zucchini slices, bell pepper pieces, and red onion chunks onto the soaked skewers, alternating between ingredients.
4. Brush the turmeric marinade over the skewers, ensuring even coating.
5. Place the skewers on the preheated grill and cook for 10-12 minutes, turning occasionally, until the chicken is cooked through and the vegetables are tender.
6. Optional: Garnish with fresh herbs like parsley or cilantro.
7. Serve these turmeric chicken and vegetable skewers as a flavorful and easy-to-make lunch.

CHAPTER 5: SNACKS AND DESSERTS

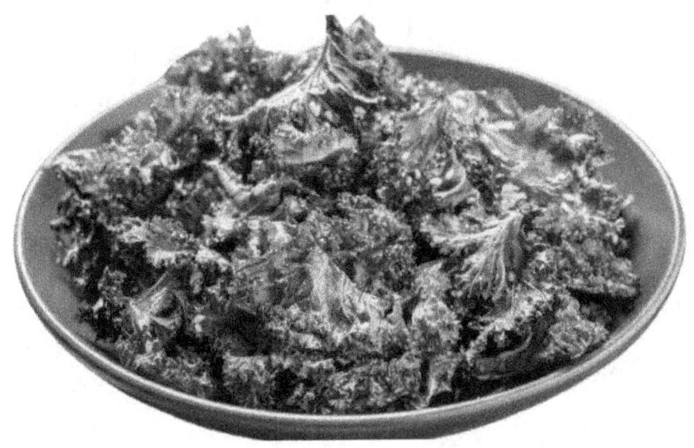

Baked Kale Chips

Ingredients:

- 1 bunch of kale, washed and thoroughly dried
- 1-2 tablespoons olive oil
- Salt to taste
- Optional: Seasonings like garlic powder, paprika, or nutritional yeast

Directions:

1. Preheat your oven to 350°F (175°C).
2. Remove the tough stems from the kale leaves and tear the leaves into bite-sized pieces.

3. In a large bowl, toss the kale pieces with olive oil. Ensure each piece is lightly coated but not drenched.

4. Arrange the kale pieces in a single layer on a baking sheet. Avoid overcrowding to allow for even baking.

5. Sprinkle salt over the kale chips. Optionally, add seasonings like garlic powder, paprika, or nutritional yeast for added flavor.

6. Bake in the preheated oven for 10-15 minutes or until the edges are crisp and the kale is no longer soggy. Keep a close eye to prevent burning.

7. Remove the kale chips from the oven and let them cool on the baking sheet for a few minutes. They will continue to crisp up as they cool.

8. Transfer the kale chips to a serving bowl and enjoy as a healthy and crunchy snack!

Avocado and Tomato Rice Cakes

Ingredients:

- 2 brown rice cakes
- 1 ripe avocado, mashed
- 1 medium tomato, diced
- 1 tablespoon lemon juice
- 1 teaspoon olive oil

- Fresh basil leaves for garnish
- Salt and pepper to taste

Directions:

1. Spread the mashed avocado evenly over each brown rice cake.
2. In a bowl, mix diced tomato with lemon juice, olive oil, salt, and pepper.
3. Spoon the tomato mixture over the avocado-covered rice cakes.
4. Garnish with fresh basil leaves for added flavor.
5. Serve these avocado and tomato rice cakes as a quick and easy-to-make snack.

Cucumber and Hummus Bites

Ingredients:

- 1 large cucumber, sliced into rounds
- 1/2 cup hummus (choose a variety without added avoids)
- Cherry tomatoes, halved, for topping
- Fresh dill or parsley for garnish
- Black pepper to taste

Directions:

1. Lay out the cucumber rounds on a serving platter or plate.

2.   Spoon a small amount of hummus onto each cucumber round.

3.   Top each cucumber and hummus bite with a halved cherry tomato.

4.   Sprinkle with black pepper for added flavor.

5.   Garnish with fresh dill or parsley.

6.   Serve these cucumber and hummus bites as a light and easy-to-make snack.

Egg and Avocado Rice Cake Stack

Ingredients:

- 2 brown rice cakes
- 2 hard-boiled eggs, sliced
- 1 ripe avocado, mashed
- Cherry tomatoes, halved, for topping
- Fresh chives or green onions, chopped
- Salt and pepper to taste

Directions:

1.   Place the brown rice cakes on a serving plate.

2.   Spread a layer of mashed avocado evenly over each rice cake.

3.   Arrange slices of hard-boiled egg on top of the avocado.

4.   Add halved cherry tomatoes on the egg slices.

5. Sprinkle chopped fresh chives or green onions over the stack.

6. Season with salt and pepper to taste.

7. Serve these egg and avocado rice cake stacks as a protein-rich and easy-to-make snack.

Nut Butter Energy Balls

Ingredients:

- 1 cup old-fashioned oats
- 1/2 cup nut butter (almond, peanut, or cashew)
- 1/3 cup honey or maple syrup
- 1/2 cup ground flaxseed
- 1/2 cup dark chocolate chips (optional)
- 1 teaspoon vanilla extract
- Pinch of salt

Directions:

1. In a large mixing bowl, combine the oats, nut butter, honey (or maple syrup), ground flaxseed, chocolate chips (if using), vanilla extract, and a pinch of salt.

2. Mix the ingredients thoroughly until well combined. If the mixture seems too dry, you can add a bit more nut butter or honey to achieve a sticky consistency.

3. Cover the bowl and refrigerate the mixture for about 30 minutes. Chilling will make it easier to form the energy balls.

4. After refrigerating, take small portions of the mixture and roll them into bite-sized balls using your hands. The size is up to your preference.

5. Place the energy balls on a parchment paper-lined tray and refrigerate for an additional 15-30 minutes to firm up.

6. Once the energy balls have set, transfer them to an airtight container and store in the refrigerator for freshness.

7. Enjoy these nutrient-packed nut butter energy balls as a quick and satisfying snack or energy boost during the day!

Apple and Almond Butter Slices

Ingredients:

- 1 apple, cored and sliced into thin rounds
- 2 tablespoons almond butter (unsweetened)
- 1 tablespoon chia seeds
- Cinnamon for sprinkling (optional)
- Drizzle of honey (optional)

Directions:

1. Arrange the apple slices on a plate.

2. Spread a thin layer of almond butter on each apple slice.

3. Sprinkle chia seeds over the almond butter.

4. Optional: Lightly dust the slices with cinnamon for extra flavor.

5. Drizzle honey over the top if desired, for a touch of sweetness.

6. Serve these apple and almond butter slices as a crunchy and easy-to-make snack.

Carrot and Hummus Roll-Ups

Ingredients:

- 2 large carrots, peeled
- 1/4 cup hummus (choose a variety without added avoids)
- Fresh parsley leaves, chopped
- Ground black pepper to taste

Directions:

1. Use a vegetable peeler to create thin, wide strips from the peeled carrots.

2. Spread a thin layer of hummus onto each carrot strip.

3. Sprinkle chopped fresh parsley over the hummus.

4. Add a dash of ground black pepper for extra flavor.

5. Carefully roll up each carrot strip with the hummus and parsley inside.

6. Secure with toothpicks if needed.

7. Serve these carrot and hummus roll-ups as a crunchy and easy-to-make snack.

Tuna and Avocado Cucumber Bites

Ingredients:

- 1 cucumber, sliced into rounds
- 1 can (5 oz) tuna in water, drained
- 1/2 avocado, mashed
- 1 tablespoon lemon juice
- Cherry tomatoes, halved, for topping
- Fresh dill or parsley for garnish
- Salt and pepper to taste

Directions:

1. Place the cucumber rounds on a serving plate.

2. In a bowl, mix the drained tuna, mashed avocado, lemon juice, salt, and pepper.

3. Spoon a small amount of the tuna and avocado mixture onto each cucumber round.

4. Top each bite with a halved cherry tomato.

5. Garnish with fresh dill or parsley for added flavor.

6. Serve these tuna and avocado cucumber bites as a protein-rich and easy-to-make snack.

Stuffed Bell Pepper Rings

Ingredients:

- 2 bell peppers (any color), sliced into rings
- 1/2 cup cottage cheese
- 1/4 cup diced cucumber
- 1/4 cup cherry tomatoes, halved
- 1 tablespoon fresh basil, chopped
- 1 teaspoon olive oil
- Salt and pepper to taste

Directions:

1. In a bowl, mix cottage cheese, diced cucumber, cherry tomatoes, chopped basil, olive oil, salt, and pepper.
2. Lay out the bell pepper rings on a serving plate.
3. Spoon the cottage cheese mixture into each bell pepper ring, filling them generously.
4. Optional: Drizzle a little extra olive oil over the top for added flavor.
5. Serve these stuffed bell pepper rings as a refreshing and easy-to-make snack.

Cucumber and Smoked Salmon Roll-Ups

Ingredients:

- 1 large cucumber, thinly sliced lengthwise
- 4 oz smoked salmon
- 1/4 cup whipped cream cheese (or a dairy-free alternative)
- 1 tablespoon capers
- Fresh dill for garnish

Directions:

1. Lay out the cucumber slices on a clean surface.
2. Spread a thin layer of whipped cream cheese over each cucumber slice.
3. Place a slice of smoked salmon on top of the cream cheese-covered cucumber.
4. Sprinkle capers evenly over the salmon.
5. Carefully roll up each cucumber slice with the salmon and cream cheese inside.
6. Secure with toothpicks if needed.
7. Garnish with fresh dill for added flavor.
8. Serve these cucumber and smoked salmon roll-ups as a protein-rich and easy-to-make snack.

Sweet Potato and Almond Butter Bites

Ingredients:

- 1 medium sweet potato, cooked and sliced into rounds
- 2 tablespoons almond butter (unsweetened)
- 1 tablespoon honey (optional)
- 1 tablespoon chopped almonds
- Cinnamon for sprinkling

Directions:

1. Lay out the sweet potato rounds on a serving plate.
2. Spread a thin layer of almond butter over each sweet potato round.
3. Drizzle honey over the almond butter if desired, for sweetness.
4. Sprinkle chopped almonds evenly over the bites.
5. Finish with a dash of cinnamon for added flavor.
6. Serve these sweet potato and almond butter bites as a nutritious and easy-to-make snack.

Cherry Tomato and Goat Cheese Stuffed Celery Sticks

Ingredients:

- 4 celery sticks, cut into manageable lengths
- 1/2 cup cherry tomatoes, halved

- 2 oz goat cheese, crumbled

- Fresh basil leaves, torn

- Olive oil for drizzling

- Balsamic glaze for drizzling (optional)

- Salt and pepper to taste

Directions:

1. In each celery stick, spread a small amount of crumbled goat cheese.

2. Top the goat cheese with halved cherry tomatoes.

3. Sprinkle torn basil leaves over the tomatoes.

4. Drizzle olive oil over the stuffed celery sticks.

5. Optional: Drizzle balsamic glaze for an extra layer of flavor.

6. Season with salt and pepper to taste.

7. Serve these cherry tomato and goat cheese stuffed celery sticks as a refreshing and easy-to-make snack.

Pomegranate and Cottage Cheese Parfait

Ingredients:

- 1 cup cottage cheese

- 1/2 cup pomegranate seeds

- 2 tablespoons chopped walnuts

- 1 teaspoon honey (optional)

- Fresh mint leaves for garnish

Directions:

1. In a glass or bowl, layer half of the cottage cheese at the bottom.

2. Add a layer of pomegranate seeds on top of the cottage cheese.

3. Sprinkle chopped walnuts over the pomegranate layer.

4. Drizzle honey over the top if desired, for sweetness.

5. Add the remaining cottage cheese as the next layer.

6. Top with the remaining pomegranate seeds.

7. Garnish with fresh mint leaves for a burst of freshness.

8. Serve this pomegranate and cottage cheese parfait as a light and easy-to-make snack.

Cinnamon Baked Pears

Ingredients:

- 2 ripe pears, halved and cored
- 2 tablespoons almond butter (unsweetened)
- 1 tablespoon chopped walnuts
- 1 teaspoon ground cinnamon
- 1 teaspoon honey (optional)
- Fresh lemon juice

Directions:

1. Preheat the oven to 375°F (190°C).

2. Place the pear halves on a baking sheet, cut side up.

3. Drizzle a bit of fresh lemon juice over each pear half to prevent browning.

4. In a small bowl, mix almond butter, chopped walnuts, and cinnamon.

5. Spoon the almond butter mixture into the center of each pear half.

6. Optional: Drizzle honey over the top for added sweetness.

7. Bake in the preheated oven for about 15-20 minutes or until the pears are tender.

8. Remove from the oven and let them cool slightly.

9. Serve these cinnamon baked pears as a warm and easy-to-make dessert.

Cocoa-Coconut Energy Bites

Ingredients:

- 1 cup rolled oats
- 1/2 cup almond butter (unsweetened)
- 1/4 cup shredded coconut (unsweetened)
- 2 tablespoons cocoa powder (unsweetened)
- 2 tablespoons honey or maple syrup
- 1 teaspoon vanilla extract
- A pinch of sea salt
- Additional shredded coconut for coating (optional)

Directions:

1. In a food processor, combine rolled oats, almond butter, shredded coconut, cocoa powder, honey or maple syrup, vanilla extract, and a pinch of sea salt.

2. Process the mixture until well combined and forms a dough-like consistency.

3. Scoop out small portions and roll them into bite-sized balls.

4. Optional: Roll the energy bites in additional shredded coconut for coating.

5. Place the energy bites on a plate or tray and refrigerate for at least 30 minutes to firm up.

6. Once firm, these cocoa-coconut energy bites are ready to serve.

Baked Apple Slices with Almond Date Crumble

Ingredients:

- 2 apples, cored and thinly sliced
- 1/4 cup almond meal
- 2 tablespoons chopped dates
- 1 tablespoon coconut oil, melted
- 1/2 teaspoon ground cinnamon
- 1/4 teaspoon nutmeg

- A pinch of sea salt

Directions:

1. Preheat the oven to 375°F (190°C).

2. In a bowl, combine almond meal, chopped dates, melted coconut oil, cinnamon, nutmeg, and a pinch of sea salt to create the crumble mixture.

3. Place the apple slices in a baking dish.

4. Sprinkle the almond date crumble evenly over the apple slices.

5. Bake in the preheated oven for about 15-20 minutes or until the apples are tender and the crumble is golden.

6. Remove from the oven and let it cool for a few minutes.

7. Serve these baked apple slices with almond date crumble as a warm and easy-to-make dessert.

Vanilla Coconut Chia Pudding

Ingredients:

- 1/4 cup chia seeds
- 1 cup coconut milk (unsweetened)
- 1 teaspoon vanilla extract
- 1 tablespoon honey or maple syrup (optional, adjust to taste)
- Sliced strawberries for topping
- Unsweetened shredded coconut for garnish

Directions:

1. In a bowl, mix chia seeds, coconut milk, vanilla extract, and honey or maple syrup (if using).

2. Whisk the mixture well and let it sit for about 5 minutes.

3. Stir the mixture again to avoid clumping, cover, and refrigerate for at least 2 hours or until it thickens.

4. Once the chia pudding has set, give it a good stir.

5. Spoon the chia pudding into serving bowls.

6. Top with sliced strawberries and sprinkle unsweetened shredded coconut over the top.

7. Optional: Drizzle a little extra honey or maple syrup for added sweetness.

8. Serve this vanilla coconut chia pudding as a light and easy-to-make dessert.

Pistachio Banana Ice Cream

Ingredients:

- 2 ripe bananas, sliced and frozen
- 1/4 cup shelled pistachios
- 1 tablespoon almond milk (unsweetened)
- 1 teaspoon vanilla extract
- A pinch of sea salt
- Chopped pistachios for topping

Directions:

1. In a blender or food processor, combine frozen banana slices, shelled pistachios, almond milk, vanilla extract, and a pinch of sea salt.
2. Blend until the mixture reaches a smooth and creamy consistency.
3. Optional: Add more almond milk if needed to achieve the desired texture.
4. Scoop the pistachio banana ice cream into serving bowls.
5. Top with chopped pistachios for added crunch.
6. Serve this pistachio banana ice cream as a refreshing and easy-to-make dessert.

Maple Pecan Baked Apples

Ingredients:

- 2 apples, cored and halved
- 2 tablespoons chopped pecans
- 1 tablespoon coconut oil, melted
- 1 tablespoon maple syrup
- 1/2 teaspoon ground cinnamon
- A pinch of sea salt

Directions:

1. Preheat the oven to 375°F (190°C).

2. In a small bowl, mix chopped pecans, melted coconut oil, maple syrup, ground cinnamon, and a pinch of sea salt.

3. Place the apple halves in a baking dish.

4. Spoon the pecan mixture evenly over the apple halves.

5. Bake in the preheated oven for about 20-25 minutes or until the apples are tender.

6. Remove from the oven and let them cool slightly.

7. Serve these maple pecan baked apples as a warm and easy-to-make dessert.

Cinnamon Pear Yogurt Parfait

Ingredients:

- 1 ripe pear, diced
- 1 cup Greek yogurt (unsweetened)
- 1 tablespoon honey or maple syrup (optional, adjust to taste)
- 1/2 teaspoon ground cinnamon
- 2 tablespoons chopped walnuts
- Fresh mint leaves for garnish

Directions:

1. In a bowl, mix diced pear with ground cinnamon.

2. In a serving glass or bowl, layer Greek yogurt, followed by the cinnamon-infused diced pear.

3. Repeat the layers until the glass is filled.

4. Optional: Drizzle honey or maple syrup over the layers for added sweetness.

5. Top the parfait with chopped walnuts and garnish with fresh mint leaves.

6. Serve this cinnamon pear yogurt parfait as a light and easy-to-make dessert.

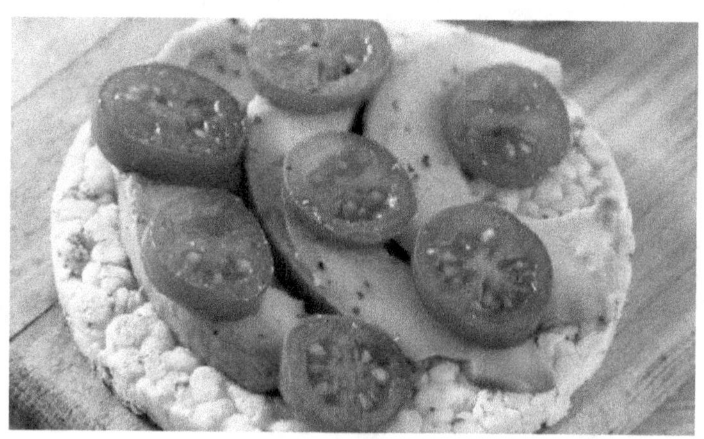

CHAPTER 6: DINNER

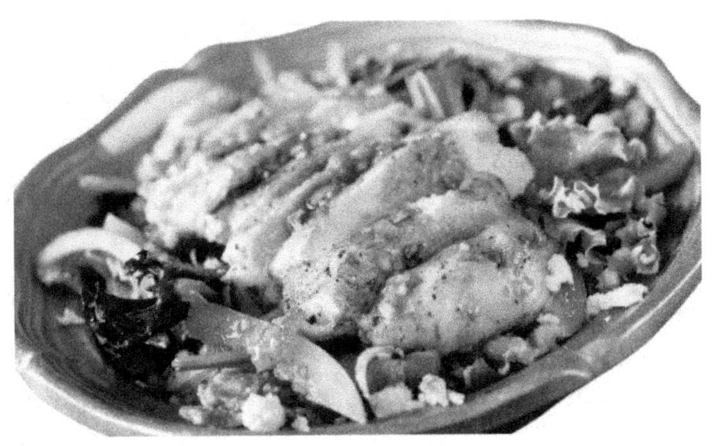

Lemon Herb Baked Chicken

Ingredients:

- 4 boneless, skinless chicken breasts
- Juice of 2 lemons
- 2 tablespoons olive oil
- 2 cloves garlic, minced
- 1 teaspoon dried thyme
- 1 teaspoon dried rosemary
- Salt and pepper to taste
- Lemon slices for garnish
- Fresh parsley for garnish

Directions:

1. Preheat the oven to 400°F (200°C).

2. In a bowl, whisk together lemon juice, olive oil, minced garlic, dried thyme, dried rosemary, salt, and pepper.

3. Place the chicken breasts in a baking dish.

4. Pour the lemon herb mixture over the chicken, ensuring even coating.

5. Optional: Marinate the chicken for 15-20 minutes for enhanced flavor.

6. Bake in the preheated oven for 25-30 minutes or until the chicken is cooked through and juices run clear.

7. Garnish with lemon slices and fresh parsley before serving.

Vegetarian Lentil and Sweet Potato Curry

Ingredients:

- 1 cup dry green or brown lentils, rinsed
- 2 sweet potatoes, peeled and diced
- 1 tablespoon coconut oil
- 1 onion, finely chopped
- 2 cloves garlic, minced
- 1 tablespoon curry powder
- 1 teaspoon ground cumin
- 1 teaspoon ground coriander
- 1 can (14 oz) diced tomatoes (unsweetened)
- 1 can (14 oz) coconut milk (unsweetened)

- Salt and pepper to taste
- Fresh cilantro for garnish
- Cooked brown rice for serving

Directions:

1. In a pot, combine lentils, sweet potatoes, and enough water to cover. Bring to a boil, then reduce heat and simmer until lentils and sweet potatoes are tender (about 20-25 minutes).
2. In a separate large skillet, heat coconut oil over medium heat. Add chopped onion and sauté until softened.
3. Add minced garlic, curry powder, ground cumin, and ground coriander to the skillet. Stir well to combine the spices with the onions.
4. Pour in diced tomatoes and coconut milk. Simmer for 10-15 minutes, allowing flavors to meld.
5. Combine the cooked lentils and sweet potatoes with the tomato-coconut mixture. Season with salt and pepper to taste.
6. Simmer for an additional 10 minutes to ensure everything is heated through and flavors meld.
7. Serve the Vegetarian Lentil and Sweet Potato Curry over cooked brown rice, garnished with fresh cilantro.

Zucchini Noodles with Pesto and Cherry Tomatoes

Ingredients:

- 4 medium-sized zucchinis, spiralized into noodles
- 1 cup cherry tomatoes, halved
- 1/2 cup pine nuts
- 2 cups fresh basil leaves
- 2 cloves garlic, minced
- 1/2 cup extra virgin olive oil
- 1/2 cup grated Parmesan cheese (optional)
- Salt and pepper to taste
- Lemon wedges for serving

Directions:

1. In a dry skillet, lightly toast pine nuts over medium heat until golden brown. Set aside to cool.
2. In a food processor, combine basil, minced garlic, and toasted pine nuts. Pulse until finely chopped.
3. With the food processor running, slowly pour in the olive oil until the mixture forms a smooth pesto.
4. If using, add grated Parmesan cheese to the pesto and pulse until well combined. Season with salt and pepper to taste.
5. In a large bowl, toss zucchini noodles with the pesto until evenly coated.

6. Gently fold in the halved cherry tomatoes.

7. Serve the Zucchini Noodles with Pesto and Cherry Tomatoes on plates, garnished with additional pine nuts and lemon wedges.

Baked Lemon Garlic Herb Chicken Thighs

Ingredients:

- 4 bone-in, skin-on chicken thighs
- Juice of 2 lemons
- 3 tablespoons olive oil
- 3 cloves garlic, minced
- 1 teaspoon dried thyme
- 1 teaspoon dried rosemary
- Salt and pepper to taste
- Lemon slices for garnish
- Fresh parsley for garnish

Directions:

1. Preheat the oven to 400°F (200°C).

2. In a bowl, whisk together lemon juice, olive oil, minced garlic, dried thyme, dried rosemary, salt, and pepper.

3. Place the chicken thighs in a baking dish.

4. Pour the lemon garlic herb mixture over the chicken, ensuring even coating.

5. Optional: Marinate the chicken for 15-20 minutes for enhanced flavor.

6. Bake in the preheated oven for 30-35 minutes or until the chicken is cooked through and the skin is crispy.

7. Garnish with lemon slices and fresh parsley before serving.

Eggplant and Chickpea Curry

Ingredients:

- 1 large eggplant, diced
- 1 can (15 oz) chickpeas, drained and rinsed
- 1 onion, finely chopped
- 2 cloves garlic, minced
- 1 tablespoon curry powder
- 1 teaspoon ground cumin
- 1 teaspoon ground coriander
- 1 can (14 oz) diced tomatoes (unsweetened)
- 1 can (14 oz) coconut milk (unsweetened)
- 1 tablespoon olive oil
- Salt and pepper to taste
- Fresh cilantro for garnish
- Cooked brown rice for serving

Directions:

1. In a large skillet, heat olive oil over medium heat. Add chopped onion and sauté until softened.

2. Add minced garlic, curry powder, ground cumin, and ground coriander to the skillet. Stir well to combine the spices.

3. Add diced eggplant to the skillet and cook until it starts to soften.

4. Pour in diced tomatoes and coconut milk. Simmer for 15-20 minutes, allowing flavors to meld.

5. Stir in chickpeas and continue simmering until the chickpeas are heated through.

6. Season the mixture with salt and pepper to taste.

7. Serve the Eggplant and Chickpea Curry over cooked brown rice, garnished with fresh cilantro.

Lemon Herb Baked Cod

Ingredients:

- 4 cod filets
- Juice of 2 lemons
- 3 tablespoons olive oil
- 2 cloves garlic, minced
- 1 teaspoon dried oregano
- 1 teaspoon dried thyme

- Salt and pepper to taste

- Lemon slices for garnish

- Fresh parsley for garnish

Directions:

1. Preheat the oven to 375°F (190°C).

2. In a bowl, whisk together lemon juice, olive oil, minced garlic, dried oregano, dried thyme, salt, and pepper.

3. Place the cod filets in a baking dish.

4. Pour the lemon herb mixture over the cod, ensuring even coating.

5. Optional: Marinate the cod for 15-20 minutes for enhanced flavor.

6. Bake in the preheated oven for 20-25 minutes or until the cod is cooked through and flakes easily.

7. Garnish with lemon slices and fresh parsley before serving.

Chickpea and Vegetable Curry

Ingredients:

- 1 can (15 oz) chickpeas, drained and rinsed

- 1 tablespoon olive oil

- 1 onion, finely chopped

- 2 bell peppers, diced (use a mix of colors)

- 1 cup cherry tomatoes, halved

- 1 zucchini, diced
- 3 cloves garlic, minced
- 1 tablespoon curry powder
- 1 teaspoon ground turmeric
- 1 teaspoon ground cumin
- 1 can (14 oz) coconut milk (unsweetened)
- Salt and pepper to taste
- Fresh cilantro for garnish
- Cooked brown rice for serving

Directions:

1. In a large skillet, heat olive oil over medium heat. Add chopped onion and sauté until softened.

2. Add minced garlic, curry powder, ground turmeric, and ground cumin to the skillet. Stir well to combine the spices.

3. Add diced bell peppers, cherry tomatoes, and zucchini. Cook until the vegetables are slightly tender.

4. Pour in the coconut milk and add chickpeas to the skillet. Simmer for 10-15 minutes until the flavors meld and the curry thickens slightly.

5. Season the mixture with salt and pepper to taste.

6. Serve the Chickpea and Vegetable Curry over cooked brown rice.

7. Garnish with fresh cilantro before serving.

Mediterranean Quinoa Salad with Grilled Chicken

Ingredients:

- 1 cup quinoa, rinsed
- 2 cups water or vegetable broth
- 4 boneless, skinless chicken breasts
- 2 tablespoons olive oil
- Juice of 1 lemon
- 1 teaspoon dried oregano
- Salt and pepper to taste
- 1 cucumber, diced
- 1 cup cherry tomatoes, halved
- 1/2 red onion, finely chopped
- 1/2 cup Kalamata olives, sliced
- 1/2 cup crumbled feta cheese
- Fresh parsley for garnish

Directions:

1. In a saucepan, bring water or vegetable broth to a boil. Add quinoa, reduce heat, cover, and simmer for 15-20 minutes or until quinoa is cooked and liquid is absorbed.
2. Preheat the grill or grill pan.
3. In a bowl, whisk together olive oil, lemon juice, dried oregano, salt, and pepper.

4. Brush the chicken breasts with the lemon-oregano mixture and grill for 6-8 minutes per side or until cooked through.

5. In a large bowl, combine cooked quinoa, diced cucumber, cherry tomatoes, chopped red onion, sliced Kalamata olives, and crumbled feta cheese.

6. Slice the grilled chicken and place it on top of the quinoa salad.

7. Garnish with fresh parsley before serving.

Salmon and Vegetable Foil Packets

Ingredients:

- 4 salmon filets
- 2 tablespoons olive oil
- Juice of 1 lemon
- 2 teaspoons Dijon mustard
- 1 teaspoon dried dill
- Salt and pepper to taste
- 2 zucchinis, thinly sliced
- 1 bell pepper, thinly sliced
- 1 cup cherry tomatoes, halved
- 4 green onions, chopped
- 4 sheets of aluminum foil

Directions:

1. Preheat the oven to 400°F (200°C).
2. In a bowl, whisk together olive oil, lemon juice, Dijon mustard, dried dill, salt, and pepper.
3. Place each salmon filet on a separate sheet of aluminum foil.
4. Brush the salmon filets with the lemon-dill mixture.
5. In a bowl, toss together zucchini slices, bell pepper slices, cherry tomatoes, and chopped green onions.
6. Divide the vegetable mixture equally among the foil packets, arranging it around the salmon.
7. Fold and seal the foil packets, creating a tight seal.
8. Place the foil packets on a baking sheet and bake in the preheated oven for 20-25 minutes or until the salmon is cooked through and the vegetables are tender.
9. Carefully open the foil packets, and serve the salmon and vegetables directly from them.

Stir-Fried Tofu with Broccoli and Cashews

Ingredients:

- 1 block extra-firm tofu, pressed and cubed
- 2 tablespoons soy sauce (low-sodium)
- 1 tablespoon rice vinegar
- 1 tablespoon hoisin sauce

- 1 tablespoon sesame oil
- 1 tablespoon olive oil
- 2 cloves garlic, minced
- 1 tablespoon fresh ginger, grated
- 2 cups broccoli florets
- 1/2 cup unsalted cashews
- Green onions, sliced, for garnish
- Cooked brown rice for serving

Directions:

1. In a bowl, combine cubed tofu with soy sauce, rice vinegar, and hoisin sauce. Allow it to marinate for at least 15 minutes.

2. Heat olive oil and sesame oil in a wok or large skillet over medium-high heat.

3. Add minced garlic and grated ginger, sauté for 1-2 minutes until fragrant.

4. Add marinated tofu to the wok and stir-fry until golden brown on all sides.

5. Toss in broccoli florets and cashews, continue stir-frying until broccoli is tender-crisp.

6. Adjust the seasoning with additional soy sauce or hoisin sauce if needed.

7. Serve the stir-fried tofu, broccoli, and cashews over cooked brown rice.

8. Garnish with sliced green onions before serving.

Lemon Garlic Shrimp with Quinoa

Ingredients:

- 1 cup quinoa, rinsed
- 2 cups vegetable broth (low-sodium)
- 1 pound large shrimp, peeled and deveined
- 2 tablespoons olive oil
- 3 cloves garlic, minced
- Zest of 1 lemon
- Juice of 1 lemon
- 1 teaspoon dried thyme
- Salt and pepper to taste
- 1 cup cherry tomatoes, halved
- Fresh parsley for garnish

Directions:

1. In a saucepan, bring vegetable broth to a boil. Add quinoa, reduce heat, cover, and simmer for 15-20 minutes or until quinoa is cooked and liquid is absorbed.
2. In a large skillet, heat olive oil over medium heat.
3. Add minced garlic to the skillet and sauté for 1-2 minutes until fragrant.
4. Add shrimp to the skillet, cooking for 2-3 minutes on each side or until they turn pink.

5. Stir in lemon zest, lemon juice, dried thyme, salt, and pepper. Cook for an additional 2 minutes.

6. Toss in cherry tomatoes and cook for another 2 minutes until they soften slightly.

7. Serve the lemon garlic shrimp over a bed of cooked quinoa.

8. Garnish with fresh parsley before serving.

Grilled Turkey and Vegetable Skewers

Ingredients:

- 1 pound lean turkey breast, cut into cubes
- 2 tablespoons olive oil
- 2 tablespoons balsamic vinegar
- 1 teaspoon dried rosemary
- 1 teaspoon dried thyme
- 2 cloves garlic, minced
- Salt and pepper to taste
- 1 zucchini, sliced
- 1 red onion, cut into chunks
- 1 bell pepper, diced
- Cherry tomatoes
- Wooden skewers, soaked in water

1. In a bowl, mix olive oil, balsamic vinegar, dried rosemary, dried thyme, minced garlic, salt, and pepper to create the marinade.
2. Add turkey cubes to the marinade, ensuring they are well-coated. Let it marinate for at least 30 minutes.
3. Preheat the grill or grill pan.
4. Thread marinated turkey, zucchini slices, red onion chunks, bell pepper, and cherry tomatoes onto the soaked wooden skewers.
5. Grill the skewers for 8-10 minutes, turning occasionally, until the turkey is cooked through and vegetables are slightly charred.
6. Serve the Grilled Turkey and Vegetable Skewers with a side of steamed quinoa or your preferred whole grain.

Vegetarian Lentil and Spinach Stuffed Bell Peppers

Ingredients:

- 4 large bell peppers, halved and seeds removed
- 1 cup dry green lentils, rinsed
- 2 1/2 cups vegetable broth (low-sodium)
- 1 tablespoon olive oil
- 1 onion, finely chopped

- 2 cloves garlic, minced

- 1 can (14 oz) diced tomatoes, drained

- 2 cups fresh spinach, chopped

- 1 teaspoon dried oregano

- 1 teaspoon ground cumin

- Salt and pepper to taste

- 1 cup shredded mozzarella cheese (optional)

- Fresh parsley for garnish

Directions:

1. Preheat the oven to 375°F (190°C).

2. In a saucepan, combine lentils and vegetable broth. Bring to a boil, then reduce heat, cover, and simmer for 25-30 minutes or until lentils are tender and the liquid is absorbed.

3. In a large skillet, heat olive oil over medium heat. Add chopped onion and sauté until softened.

4. Add minced garlic, diced tomatoes, chopped spinach, dried oregano, ground cumin, salt, and pepper. Cook for an additional 5 minutes.

5. Combine the cooked lentils with the vegetable mixture.

6. Place the halved bell peppers in a baking dish and fill each half with the lentil and spinach mixture.

7. If desired, sprinkle shredded mozzarella cheese on top.

8. Bake in the preheated oven for 25-30 minutes or until the bell peppers are tender.

9. Garnish with fresh parsley before serving.

Turkey Stir-Fry with Bok Choy and Brown Rice Noodles

Ingredients:

- 1 lb ground turkey
- 8 oz brown rice noodles
- 1 large bok choy, chopped
- 1 red bell pepper, thinly sliced
- 2 carrots, julienned
- 3 cloves garlic, minced
- 1 tablespoon fresh ginger, grated
- 1/4 cup low-sodium soy sauce
- 2 tablespoons oyster sauce
- 1 tablespoon sesame oil
- 1 tablespoon vegetable oil
- Sesame seeds for garnish (optional)
- Green onions, chopped, for garnish (optional)

Directions:

1. Cook brown rice noodles according to package instructions. Drain and set aside.

2. In a wok or large skillet, heat vegetable oil over medium-high heat.

3. Add ground turkey to the wok and cook until browned, breaking it apart with a spoon.

4. Stir in minced garlic and grated ginger, cooking for an additional minute until fragrant.

5. Add sliced bell pepper and julienned carrots to the wok, stir-frying for 2-3 minutes until vegetables start to soften.

6. Stir in chopped bok choy and continue to cook until it wilts and becomes tender.

7. In a small bowl, mix soy sauce, oyster sauce, and sesame oil. Pour the sauce over the turkey and vegetable mixture in the wok.

8. Add the cooked brown rice noodles to the wok, tossing everything together until well coated in the sauce.

9. Continue to cook for an additional 2-3 minutes, ensuring the noodles and vegetables are heated through.

10. Garnish with sesame seeds and chopped green onions if desired.

11. Serve the turkey stir-fry with bok choy and brown rice noodles immediately. Enjoy your healthy and delicious meal!

Eggplant Lasagna with Ground Turkey and Tomato-Based Sauce

Ingredients:

- 2 large eggplants, thinly sliced lengthwise
- 1 lb ground turkey
- 1 onion, finely chopped
- 3 cloves garlic, minced
- 1 can (28 oz) crushed tomatoes
- 1 can (14 oz) diced tomatoes, drained
- 2 tablespoons tomato paste
- 1 teaspoon dried oregano
- 1 teaspoon dried basil
- 1/2 teaspoon dried thyme
- Salt and pepper to taste
- 2 cups ricotta cheese
- 1 egg
- 2 cups shredded mozzarella cheese
- 1/2 cup grated Parmesan cheese

- Fresh basil for garnish (optional)

Directions:

1. Preheat the oven to 375°F (190°C).

2. Lay out the eggplant slices on a baking sheet, sprinkle with salt, and let them sit for about 15 minutes to draw out excess moisture. Pat them dry with a paper towel.

3. In a large skillet over medium heat, cook the ground turkey until browned. Add chopped onion and minced garlic, cooking until softened.

4. Stir in crushed tomatoes, diced tomatoes, tomato paste, dried oregano, dried basil, dried thyme, salt, and pepper. Simmer the sauce for about 15-20 minutes, allowing flavors to meld.

5. In a bowl, combine ricotta cheese and an egg, mixing until well blended.

6. Grease a baking dish and begin layering: start with a layer of tomato sauce, followed by a layer of eggplant slices, a layer of ricotta mixture, and a sprinkle of mozzarella cheese. Repeat until ingredients are used up, finishing with a layer of tomato sauce on top.

7. Sprinkle grated Parmesan cheese over the final layer.

8. Cover the baking dish with foil and bake for 30 minutes. Remove the foil and bake for an additional 15-20 minutes until the top is golden and bubbly.

9. Allow the eggplant lasagna to rest for 10 minutes before slicing.

10. Garnish with fresh basil if desired and serve. Enjoy your delicious and nutritious eggplant lasagna with ground turkey!

Turkey Chili with Kidney Beans, Tomatoes, and a Variety of Spices

Ingredients:

- 1 lb ground turkey
- 1 onion, finely chopped
- 3 cloves garlic, minced
- 1 can (28 oz) crushed tomatoes
- 1 can (14 oz) diced tomatoes, undrained
- 2 cans (15 oz each) kidney beans, drained and rinsed
- 1 bell pepper, diced
- 2 tablespoons tomato paste
- 1 cup beef or vegetable broth
- 1 tablespoon chili powder
- 1 teaspoon ground cumin
- 1 teaspoon paprika
- 1/2 teaspoon dried oregano

- 1/2 teaspoon ground coriander

- 1/4 teaspoon cayenne pepper (adjust to taste)

- Salt and black pepper to taste

- Olive oil for cooking

- Optional toppings: shredded cheese, chopped green onions, sour cream

Directions:

1. In a large pot or Dutch oven, heat olive oil over medium heat. Add chopped onion and cook until softened.

2. Add minced garlic to the pot and cook for an additional minute until fragrant.

3. Add ground turkey to the pot, breaking it apart with a spoon, and cook until browned.

4. Stir in diced bell pepper and cook for 2-3 minutes until slightly softened.

5. Add crushed tomatoes, diced tomatoes, tomato paste, kidney beans, and broth to the pot. Stir well to combine.

6. Season the chili with chili powder, ground cumin, paprika, dried oregano, ground coriander, cayenne pepper, salt, and black pepper. Adjust the seasoning to your taste.

7. Bring the chili to a simmer, then reduce heat to low and let it cook uncovered for at least 30-40 minutes, allowing flavors to meld.

8. If needed, add more broth to achieve your desired consistency.

9. Serve the turkey chili hot, garnished with shredded cheese, chopped green onions, or a dollop of sour cream if desired.

10. Enjoy your hearty and flavorful turkey chili!

Grilled Portobello Mushrooms with Quinoa and Vegetable Stuffing

Ingredients:

- 4 large portobello mushrooms, stems removed
- 1 cup quinoa, rinsed
- 2 cups vegetable broth
- 1 red bell pepper, diced
- 1 zucchini, diced
- 1 cup cherry tomatoes, halved
- 1/2 cup red onion, finely chopped
- 2 cloves garlic, minced
- 1/4 cup fresh parsley, chopped

- 1/4 cup feta cheese, crumbled (optional)

- 3 tablespoons olive oil

- 1 tablespoon balsamic vinegar

- Salt and black pepper to taste

Directions:

1. Preheat the grill to medium-high heat.

2. In a saucepan, bring the vegetable broth to a boil. Add rinsed quinoa, reduce heat to low, cover, and simmer for 15-20 minutes or until quinoa is cooked and liquid is absorbed.

3. While the quinoa is cooking, brush the portobello mushrooms with olive oil and season with salt and pepper.

4. Grill the portobello mushrooms for about 4-5 minutes per side, or until they are tender and have grill marks.

5. In a large skillet, heat 1 tablespoon of olive oil over medium heat. Add diced red bell pepper, zucchini, cherry tomatoes, red onion, and minced garlic. Sauté for 5-7 minutes until vegetables are softened.

6. Fluff the cooked quinoa with a fork and add it to the skillet with the sautéed vegetables. Mix well.

7. Stir in chopped parsley, crumbled feta cheese (if using), balsamic vinegar, and the remaining olive oil. Season with salt and pepper to taste.

8. Place the grilled portobello mushrooms on a serving plate with the concave side up.

9. Spoon the quinoa and vegetable stuffing into each mushroom cap, pressing down gently.

10. Garnish with additional parsley and serve immediately.

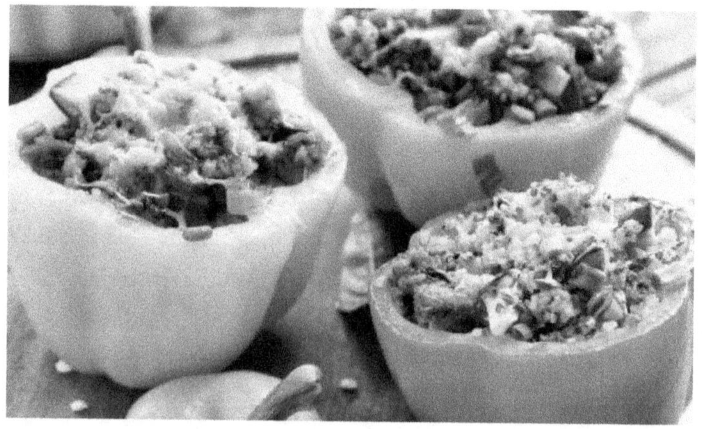

CHAPTER 7: SOUPS AND STEWS

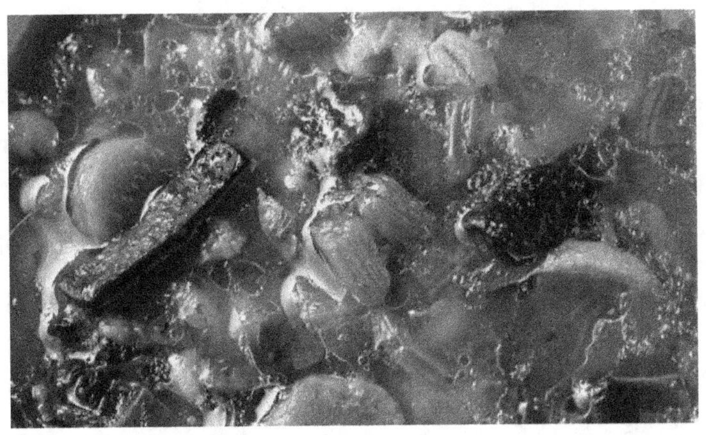

Quinoa and Kale Soup

Ingredients:

- 1 cup quinoa, rinsed
- 6 cups vegetable broth (low-sodium)
- 1 tablespoon olive oil
- 1 onion, finely chopped
- 2 carrots, diced
- 2 celery stalks, chopped
- 3 cloves garlic, minced
- 1 teaspoon dried thyme
- 1 teaspoon ground coriander
- Salt and pepper to taste
- 4 cups kale, stems removed and chopped

- Juice of 1 lemon
- Fresh parsley for garnish

Directions:

1. In a large pot, heat olive oil over medium heat. Add chopped onion, diced carrots, and chopped celery. Sauté until vegetables are softened.
2. Add minced garlic, dried thyme, ground coriander, salt, and pepper. Sauté for an additional 2 minutes until fragrant.
3. Pour in vegetable broth and bring to a boil.
4. Stir in rinsed quinoa, reduce heat to low, cover, and simmer for 15-20 minutes or until quinoa is cooked.
5. Add chopped kale to the pot and cook for an additional 5 minutes until wilted.
6. Adjust the seasoning if needed.
7. Finish by adding the juice of one lemon for a refreshing twist.
8. Serve the Quinoa and Kale Soup hot, garnished with fresh parsley.

Mushroom and Barley Soup

Ingredients:

- 1 cup pearl barley, rinsed
- 6 cups vegetable broth (low-sodium)

- 1 tablespoon olive oil

- 1 onion, finely chopped

- 2 carrots, diced

- 2 celery stalks, chopped

- 8 oz mushrooms, sliced

- 3 cloves garlic, minced

- 1 teaspoon dried thyme

- Salt and pepper to taste

- 4 cups spinach, chopped

- Juice of 1 lemon

- Fresh dill for garnish

Directions:

1. In a large pot, heat olive oil over medium heat. Add chopped onion, diced carrots, and chopped celery. Sauté until vegetables are softened.

2. Add sliced mushrooms and minced garlic. Cook for 5 minutes until mushrooms release their moisture.

3. Pour in vegetable broth and bring to a boil.

4. Stir in rinsed pearl barley, dried thyme, salt, and pepper. Reduce heat to low, cover, and simmer for 30-35 minutes or until barley is tender.

5. Add chopped spinach to the pot and cook for an additional 5 minutes until wilted.

6. Adjust the seasoning if needed.

7. Finish by adding the juice of one lemon for a bright flavor.

8. Serve the Mushroom and Barley Soup hot, garnished with fresh dill.

Coconut Chickpea Stew

Ingredients:

- 2 cans (15 oz each) chickpeas, drained and rinsed
- 1 tablespoon coconut oil
- 1 onion, finely chopped
- 3 carrots, sliced
- 2 bell peppers (any color), diced
- 3 cloves garlic, minced
- 1 can (14 oz) coconut milk (full-fat or light)
- 4 cups vegetable broth (low-sodium)
- 1 teaspoon ground turmeric
- 1 teaspoon ground coriander
- 1/2 teaspoon cayenne pepper (adjust to taste)
- Salt and pepper to taste
- Fresh cilantro for garnish

Directions:

1. In a large pot, heat coconut oil over medium heat. Add chopped onion, sliced carrots, and diced bell peppers. Sauté until softened.

2. Add minced garlic, ground turmeric, ground coriander, cayenne pepper, salt, and pepper. Sauté for an additional 2 minutes until fragrant.

3. Pour in vegetable broth and bring to a boil.

4. Stir in drained chickpeas, coconut milk, and reduce heat to low. Cover and simmer for 20-25 minutes.

5. Adjust the seasoning if needed.

6. Serve the Coconut Chickpea Stew hot, garnished with fresh cilantro.

Red Lentil and Spinach Soup

Ingredients:

- 1 cup red lentils, rinsed
- 6 cups vegetable broth (low-sodium)
- 1 tablespoon olive oil
- 1 onion, finely chopped
- 2 carrots, diced
- 2 celery stalks, chopped
- 3 cloves garlic, minced
- 1 teaspoon ground cumin
- 1 teaspoon smoked paprika
- Salt and pepper to taste
- 4 cups fresh spinach, chopped
- Juice of 1 lemon

- Fresh parsley for garnish

Directions:

1. In a large pot, heat olive oil over medium heat. Add chopped onion, diced carrots, and chopped celery. Sauté until vegetables are softened.
2. Add minced garlic, ground cumin, smoked paprika, salt, and pepper. Sauté for an additional 2 minutes until fragrant.
3. Pour in vegetable broth and bring to a boil.
4. Stir in rinsed red lentils, reduce heat to low, cover, and simmer for 15-20 minutes or until lentils are cooked.
5. Add chopped spinach to the pot and cook for an additional 5 minutes until wilted.
6. Adjust the seasoning if needed.
7. Finish by adding the juice of one lemon for a refreshing twist.
8. Serve the Red Lentil and Spinach Soup hot, garnished with fresh parsley.

Vegetable and Lentil Stew

Ingredients:

- 1 cup green or brown lentils, rinsed
- 6 cups vegetable broth (low-sodium)
- 1 tablespoon olive oil

- 1 onion, finely chopped
- 2 carrots, diced
- 2 zucchinis, sliced
- 3 cloves garlic, minced
- 1 can (14 oz) diced tomatoes, undrained
- 4 cups kale, stems removed and chopped
- 1 teaspoon dried thyme
- Salt and pepper to taste
- 1 lemon, sliced for garnish
- Fresh parsley for garnish

Directions:

1. In a large pot, heat olive oil over medium heat. Add chopped onion, diced carrots, and sliced zucchinis. Sauté until vegetables are softened.
2. Add minced garlic, dried thyme, salt, and pepper. Sauté for an additional 2 minutes until fragrant.
3. Pour in vegetable broth and bring to a boil.
4. Stir in rinsed lentils, diced tomatoes (with juice), and kale. Reduce heat to low, cover, and simmer for 20-25 minutes or until lentils are tender.
5. Adjust the seasoning if needed.
6. Serve the Vegetable and Lentil Stew hot, garnished with lemon slices and fresh parsley.

Butternut Squash and Apple Soup

Ingredients:

- 1 medium butternut squash, peeled, seeded, and diced
- 2 apples, peeled, cored, and diced
- 1 onion, finely chopped
- 2 tablespoons olive oil
- 4 cups vegetable broth (low-sodium)
- 1 teaspoon ground ginger
- 1/2 teaspoon ground cinnamon
- Salt and pepper to taste
- 1 cup coconut milk (full-fat or light)
- Toasted pumpkin seeds for garnish (optional)

Directions:

1. In a large pot, heat olive oil over medium heat. Add chopped onion and sauté until softened.
2. Add diced butternut squash and apples to the pot. Sauté for 5 minutes to enhance flavors.
3. Pour in vegetable broth and bring to a boil.
4. Stir in ground ginger, ground cinnamon, salt, and pepper. Reduce heat to low, cover, and simmer for 20-25 minutes or until squash and apples are tender.
5. Using an immersion blender, puree the soup until smooth.

6. Stir in coconut milk to add creaminess. Adjust the seasoning if needed.

7. Serve the Butternut Squash and Apple Soup hot, garnished with toasted pumpkin seeds if desired.

Cauliflower and Leek Soup

Ingredients:

- 1 head cauliflower, chopped
- 2 leeks, white and light green parts, sliced
- 1 onion, finely chopped
- 2 tablespoons olive oil
- 4 cups vegetable broth (low-sodium)
- 3 cloves garlic, minced
- 1 teaspoon ground turmeric
- 1/2 teaspoon ground cumin
- Salt and pepper to taste
- 1 can (14 oz) coconut milk (full-fat or light)
- Fresh chives for garnish

Directions:

1. In a large pot, heat olive oil over medium heat. Add chopped onion, sliced leeks, and minced garlic. Sauté until vegetables are softened.

2. Add chopped cauliflower to the pot and sauté for an additional 5 minutes.

3. Pour in vegetable broth and bring to a boil.

4. Stir in ground turmeric, ground cumin, salt, and pepper. Reduce heat to low, cover, and simmer for 20-25 minutes or until cauliflower is tender.

5. Using an immersion blender, puree the soup until smooth.

6. Stir in coconut milk to add creaminess. Adjust the seasoning if needed.

7. Serve the Cauliflower and Leek Soup hot, garnished with fresh chives.

Chickpea and Spinach Stew

Ingredients:

- 2 cans (15 oz each) chickpeas, drained and rinsed
- 1 onion, finely chopped
- 3 cloves garlic, minced
- 2 tablespoons olive oil
- 1 can (14 oz) diced tomatoes, undrained
- 4 cups vegetable broth (low-sodium)
- 1 teaspoon ground cumin
- 1 teaspoon smoked paprika
- Salt and pepper to taste
- 4 cups fresh spinach, chopped
- Juice of 1 lemon

- Fresh cilantro for garnish

Directions:

1. In a large pot, heat olive oil over medium heat. Add chopped onion and sauté until softened.

2. Add minced garlic and cook for an additional 2 minutes until fragrant.

3. Add chickpeas, diced tomatoes (with juice), ground cumin, smoked paprika, salt, and pepper. Stir well.

4. Pour in vegetable broth and bring to a boil.

5. Reduce heat to low, cover, and simmer for 15-20 minutes to allow flavors to meld.

6. Stir in fresh chopped spinach and cook until wilted.

7. Adjust the seasoning if needed.

8. Finish by adding the juice of one lemon for a hint of citrus freshness.

9. Serve the Chickpea and Spinach Stew hot, garnished with fresh cilantro.

Lentil and Vegetable Soup

Ingredients:

- 1 cup dry green or brown lentils, rinsed
- 1 onion, finely chopped
- 2 carrots, diced
- 2 celery stalks, chopped

- 3 cloves garlic, minced
- 2 tablespoons olive oil
- 6 cups vegetable broth (low-sodium)
- 1 can (14 oz) diced tomatoes, undrained
- 1 teaspoon ground coriander
- 1 teaspoon ground cumin
- Salt and pepper to taste
- 4 cups kale, stems removed and chopped
- Juice of 1 lemon
- Fresh parsley for garnish

Directions:

1. In a large pot, heat olive oil over medium heat. Add chopped onion, diced carrots, chopped celery, and minced garlic. Sauté until vegetables are softened.
2. Add rinsed lentils to the pot and stir well.
3. Pour in vegetable broth and bring to a boil.
4. Stir in diced tomatoes (with juice), ground coriander, ground cumin, salt, and pepper. Reduce heat to low, cover, and simmer for 25-30 minutes or until lentils are tender.
5. Add chopped kale to the pot and cook for an additional 5 minutes until wilted.
6. Adjust the seasoning if needed.

7. Finish by adding the juice of one lemon for a refreshing kick.

8. Serve the Lentil and Vegetable Soup hot, garnished with fresh parsley.

Mushroom and Wild Rice Soup

Ingredients:

- 1 cup wild rice, cooked
- 1 onion, finely chopped
- 2 celery stalks, diced
- 2 carrots, sliced
- 8 oz cremini mushrooms, sliced
- 3 cloves garlic, minced
- 2 tablespoons olive oil
- 6 cups vegetable broth (low-sodium)
- 1 teaspoon dried thyme
- 1 teaspoon rosemary
- Salt and pepper to taste
- 4 cups kale, stems removed and chopped
- Juice of 1 lemon
- Fresh parsley for garnish

Directions:

1. In a large pot, heat olive oil over medium heat.

2. Add chopped onion, diced celery, sliced carrots, sliced mushrooms, and minced garlic. Sauté until vegetables are softened.

3. Pour in vegetable broth and bring to a boil.

4. Stir in cooked wild rice, dried thyme, rosemary, salt, and pepper. Reduce heat to low, cover, and simmer for 15-20 minutes.

5. Add chopped kale to the pot and cook until wilted.

6. Adjust the seasoning if needed.

7. Finish by adding the juice of one lemon for a refreshing touch.

8. Serve the Mushroom and Wild Rice Soup hot, garnished with fresh parsley.

Turmeric Cauliflower Soup

Ingredients:

- 1 large cauliflower, cut into florets
- 1 onion, chopped
- 3 cloves garlic, minced
- 1 tablespoon fresh ginger, grated
- 1 teaspoon ground turmeric
- 1/2 teaspoon ground cumin
- 1/2 teaspoon ground coriander

- 4 cups vegetable broth

- 1 can (14 oz) coconut milk

- 2 tablespoons olive oil

- Salt and black pepper to taste

- Fresh cilantro for garnish (optional)

Directions:

1. In a large pot, heat olive oil over medium heat. Add chopped onions and sauté until they become translucent.

2. Add minced garlic and grated ginger to the pot, stirring for an additional minute until fragrant.

3. Sprinkle ground turmeric, ground cumin, and ground coriander over the onion mixture. Stir well to coat the onions in the spices.

4. Add cauliflower florets to the pot and cook for about 5 minutes, allowing them to slightly brown.

5. Pour in vegetable broth, ensuring it covers the cauliflower. Bring the mixture to a boil, then reduce heat and simmer until cauliflower is tender.

6. Use an immersion blender to blend the soup until smooth. If you don't have an immersion blender, carefully transfer the soup in batches to a blender and blend until smooth.

7. Return the blended soup to the pot over low heat.

8. Stir in coconut milk, allowing it to warm through. Season with salt and black pepper to taste.

9. Simmer the soup for an additional 5-7 minutes, allowing flavors to meld.

10. Ladle the turmeric cauliflower soup into bowls, garnish with fresh cilantro if desired, and serve hot.

Bean and Kale Sausage Stew

Ingredients:

- 1 lb turkey sausage, sliced
- 1 onion, chopped
- 3 cloves garlic, minced
- 1 can (15 oz) white beans, drained and rinsed
- 1 bunch kale, stems removed and leaves chopped
- 1 can (14 oz) diced tomatoes, undrained
- 4 cups chicken or vegetable broth
- 1 teaspoon dried oregano
- 1 teaspoon dried thyme
- 1/2 teaspoon red pepper flakes (optional)
- Salt and black pepper to taste
- 2 tablespoons olive oil
- Fresh parsley for garnish (optional)

Directions:

1. In a large pot, heat olive oil over medium heat. Add sliced turkey sausage and cook until browned. Remove sausage from the pot and set aside.

2. In the same pot, add chopped onions and sauté until they become translucent.

3. Add minced garlic to the pot and cook for an additional minute until fragrant.

4. Return the cooked sausage to the pot and stir in white beans, chopped kale, diced tomatoes, oregano, thyme, and red pepper flakes (if using).

5. Pour in chicken or vegetable broth, ensuring it covers the ingredients. Bring the mixture to a simmer.

6. Reduce the heat to low, cover the pot, and let it simmer for about 20-25 minutes until kale is tender and flavors meld.

7. Season the stew with salt and black pepper to taste.

8. Serve the bean and kale sausage stew hot, garnished with fresh parsley if desired.

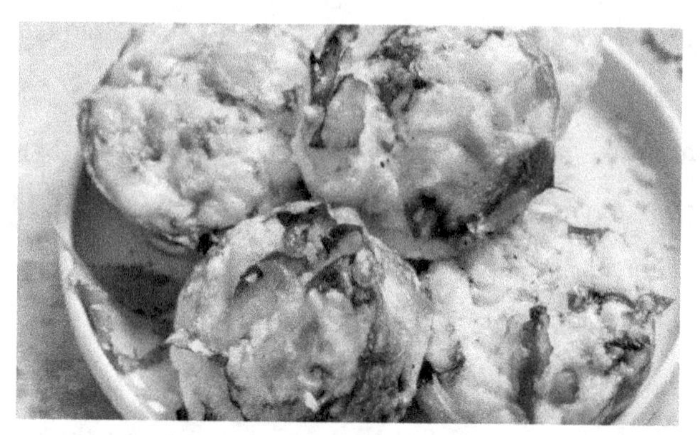

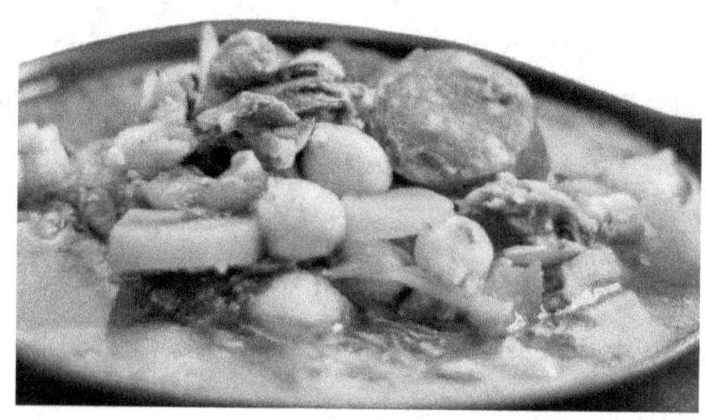

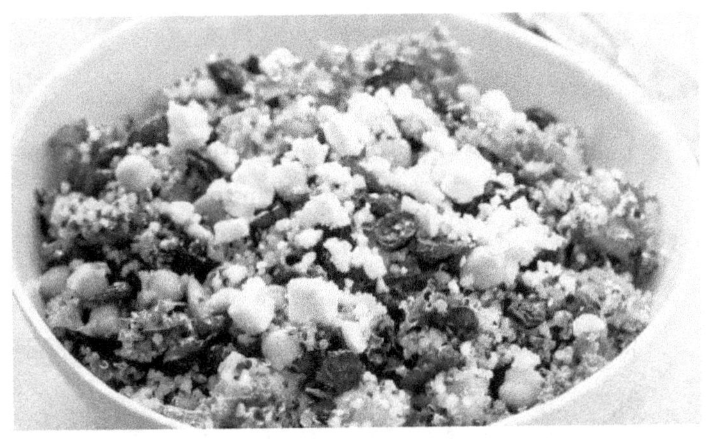

Quinoa and Chickpea Salad

Ingredients:

- 1 cup quinoa, cooked and cooled
- 1 can (14 oz) chickpeas, drained and rinsed
- 1 cucumber, diced
- 1 bell pepper (any color), diced
- 1 cup cherry tomatoes, halved
- 1/2 red onion, finely chopped
- 1/4 cup Kalamata olives, sliced
- 1/4 cup fresh parsley, chopped

For the Dressing:

- 3 tablespoons extra-virgin olive oil
- 2 tablespoons fresh lemon juice

- 1 teaspoon Dijon mustard
- 1 clove garlic, minced
- Salt and pepper to taste

Directions:

1. In a large bowl, combine the cooked quinoa, chickpeas, diced cucumber, diced bell pepper, cherry tomatoes, chopped red onion, olives, and fresh parsley.
2. In a small bowl, whisk together the olive oil, lemon juice, Dijon mustard, minced garlic, salt, and pepper to create the dressing.
3. Pour the dressing over the salad and toss gently until well combined.
4. Adjust the salt and pepper according to your taste preferences.
5. Chill the Quinoa and Chickpea Salad in the refrigerator for at least 30 minutes before serving to allow the flavors to meld.
6. Serve the salad on a bed of fresh greens or enjoy it on its own.

Spinach and Strawberry Salad with Almond Vinaigrette

Ingredients:

- 4 cups fresh baby spinach, washed

- 1 cup strawberries, hulled and sliced
- 1/4 cup sliced almonds, toasted
- 1/4 cup crumbled feta cheese (optional)

For the Almond Vinaigrette:

- 3 tablespoons almond oil
- 2 tablespoons apple cider vinegar
- 1 teaspoon honey
- 1 teaspoon Dijon mustard
- Salt and pepper to taste

Directions:

1. In a large bowl, combine fresh baby spinach, sliced strawberries, and toasted sliced almonds.
2. If desired, sprinkle crumbled feta cheese over the salad for added flavor.
3. In a small bowl, whisk together almond oil, apple cider vinegar, honey, Dijon mustard, salt, and pepper to create the almond vinaigrette.
4. Drizzle the almond vinaigrette over the salad and toss gently until well coated.
5. Adjust salt and pepper according to your taste preferences.
6. Serve the Spinach and Strawberry Salad immediately as a refreshing and nutrient-packed side dish.

Mango Avocado Quinoa Salad

Ingredients:

- 1 cup quinoa, cooked and cooled
- 1 ripe mango, peeled and diced
- 1 avocado, diced
- 1/2 red onion, finely chopped
- 1/4 cup fresh cilantro, chopped
- 1/4 cup pumpkin seeds (pepitas), toasted
- Juice of 1 lime
- Salt and pepper to taste

Directions:

1. In a large bowl, combine the cooked quinoa, diced mango, diced avocado, chopped red onion, chopped cilantro, and toasted pumpkin seeds.
2. Squeeze the juice of one lime over the ingredients to add a refreshing citrus flavor.
3. Gently toss the salad until all the ingredients are well mixed.
4. Season with salt and pepper to taste. Adjust the seasoning as needed.
5. Allow the Mango Avocado Quinoa Salad to chill in the refrigerator for about 15-20 minutes to enhance the flavors.

6. Serve the salad as a vibrant and nutrient-packed side dish.

Greek Lentil Salad

Ingredients:

- 1 cup green lentils, cooked and cooled
- 1 cucumber, diced
- 1 cup cherry tomatoes, halved
- 1/2 red onion, finely chopped
- 1/2 cup Kalamata olives, sliced
- 1/2 cup crumbled feta cheese
- 1/4 cup fresh parsley, chopped

For the Dressing:

- 3 tablespoons extra-virgin olive oil
- 2 tablespoons red wine vinegar
- 1 teaspoon dried oregano
- Salt and pepper to taste

Directions:

1. In a large bowl, combine the cooked green lentils, diced cucumber, halved cherry tomatoes, chopped red onion, sliced Kalamata olives, crumbled feta cheese, and chopped fresh parsley.

2. In a small bowl, whisk together the olive oil, red wine vinegar, dried oregano, salt, and pepper to create the dressing.

3. Drizzle the dressing over the salad and toss gently until well combined.

4. Adjust the salt and pepper according to your taste preferences.

5. Allow the Greek Lentil Salad to marinate in the refrigerator for at least 20 minutes before serving to enhance the flavors.

6. Serve the salad as a flavorful and protein-rich option!

Citrus Avocado Salad

Ingredients:

- 4 cups mixed salad greens (e.g., spinach, arugula, and watercress)
- 1 ripe avocado, sliced
- 1 orange, peeled and segmented
- 1 grapefruit, peeled and segmented
- 1/4 cup sliced almonds, toasted
- 1 tablespoon fresh mint, chopped

For the Citrus Vinaigrette:

- 3 tablespoons extra-virgin olive oil
- 2 tablespoons fresh orange juice

- 1 tablespoon fresh lemon juice

- 1 teaspoon honey

- Salt and pepper to taste

Directions:

1. In a large salad bowl, combine the mixed greens, sliced avocado, orange segments, grapefruit segments, toasted sliced almonds, and chopped fresh mint.

2. In a small bowl, whisk together the olive oil, fresh orange juice, fresh lemon juice, honey, salt, and pepper to create the citrus vinaigrette.

3. Drizzle the citrus vinaigrette over the salad and toss gently until the ingredients are well coated.

4. Adjust the salt and pepper according to your taste preferences.

5. Serve the Citrus Avocado Salad immediately as a refreshing and vitamin-packed side dish.

Apple Walnut Quinoa Salad

Ingredients:

- 1 cup cooked quinoa, cooled

- 1 apple, cored and diced (use a variety suitable for your taste)

- 1/2 cup walnuts, chopped and toasted

- 1/4 cup dried cranberries

- 1/4 cup crumbled goat cheese (optional)
- 2 tablespoons fresh chives, chopped

For the Maple Dijon Vinaigrette:

- 3 tablespoons extra-virgin olive oil
- 1 tablespoon apple cider vinegar
- 1 tablespoon pure maple syrup
- 1 teaspoon Dijon mustard
- Salt and pepper to taste

Directions:

1. In a large bowl, combine cooked quinoa, diced apple, toasted walnuts, dried cranberries, crumbled goat cheese (if using), and chopped fresh chives.

2. In a small bowl, whisk together olive oil, apple cider vinegar, maple syrup, Dijon mustard, salt, and pepper to create the Maple Dijon Vinaigrette.

3. Drizzle the vinaigrette over the salad and toss gently until all ingredients are well coated.

4. Adjust the salt and pepper according to your taste preferences.

5. Allow the Apple Walnut Quinoa Salad to rest for a few minutes to let the flavors meld.

6. Serve and enjoy the salad as a delicious and wholesome side dish!

Asian-Inspired Sesame Ginger Salad

Ingredients:

- 4 cups mixed salad greens (e.g., spinach, kale, and romaine)
- 1 cup shredded red cabbage
- 1 carrot, julienned
- 1 red bell pepper, thinly sliced
- 1/2 cup edamame, cooked and shelled
- 1/4 cup sliced almonds, toasted
- 2 tablespoons sesame seeds

For the Sesame Ginger Dressing:

- 3 tablespoons sesame oil
- 2 tablespoons rice vinegar
- 1 tablespoon soy sauce (use tamari for a gluten-free option)
- 1 tablespoon fresh ginger, grated
- 1 teaspoon honey or maple syrup
- 1 clove garlic, minced
- Salt and pepper to taste

Directions:

1. In a large salad bowl, combine mixed greens, shredded red cabbage, julienned carrot, sliced red bell pepper, cooked edamame, toasted sliced almonds, and sesame seeds.

2. In a small bowl, whisk together sesame oil, rice vinegar, soy sauce, grated fresh ginger, honey or maple syrup, minced garlic, salt, and pepper to create the Sesame Ginger Dressing.

3. Drizzle the dressing over the salad and toss gently until all ingredients are well coated.

4. Adjust the salt and pepper according to your taste preferences.

5. Allow the Asian-Inspired Sesame Ginger Salad to marinate for a few minutes to enhance the flavors.

6. Serve the salad as a flavorful and nutrient-packed option!

Roasted Beet and Goat Cheese Salad

Ingredients:

- 3 medium-sized beets, peeled and cubed
- 1 tablespoon olive oil
- Salt and pepper to taste
- 4 cups mixed salad greens (e.g., arugula, watercress, and baby spinach)
- 1/2 cup crumbled goat cheese
- 1/4 cup walnuts, toasted
- 2 tablespoons balsamic vinegar
- 2 tablespoons extra-virgin olive oil

- 1 teaspoon honey

Directions:

1. Preheat the oven to 400°F (200°C).

2. Toss the cubed beets with olive oil, salt, and pepper. Spread them on a baking sheet in a single layer.

3. Roast the beets in the preheated oven for about 25-30 minutes or until they are tender. Allow them to cool slightly.

4. In a large salad bowl, combine the mixed greens, roasted beets, crumbled goat cheese, and toasted walnuts.

5. In a small bowl, whisk together balsamic vinegar, extra-virgin olive oil, and honey to create the dressing.

6. Drizzle the dressing over the salad and toss gently until all ingredients are well coated.

7. Adjust the salt and pepper according to your taste preferences.

8. Serve and enjoy the Roasted Beet and Goat Cheese Salad!

Pomegranate and Almond Spinach Salad

Ingredients:

- 4 cups fresh baby spinach leaves
- 1 cup pomegranate arils (seeds)
- 1/2 cup sliced almonds, toasted

- 1/4 cup red onion, thinly sliced

- 1/4 cup feta cheese, crumbled (optional)

For the Citrus Vinaigrette:

- 3 tablespoons extra-virgin olive oil

- Juice of 1 orange

- Zest of 1 lemon

- 1 tablespoon balsamic vinegar

- 1 teaspoon honey

- Salt and pepper to taste

Directions:

1. In a large salad bowl, combine fresh baby spinach leaves, pomegranate arils, toasted sliced almonds, thinly sliced red onion, and crumbled feta cheese (if using).

2. In a small bowl, whisk together olive oil, orange juice, lemon zest, balsamic vinegar, honey, salt, and pepper to create the Citrus Vinaigrette.

3. Drizzle the vinaigrette over the salad and toss gently until all ingredients are well coated.

4. Adjust the salt and pepper according to your taste preferences.

5. Allow the Pomegranate and Almond Spinach Salad to sit for a few minutes to let the flavors meld.

6. Serve the salad as a refreshing and nutrient-rich option!

Quinoa and Roasted Vegetable Salad

Ingredients:

- 1 cup cooked quinoa, cooled
- 1 cup cherry tomatoes, halved
- 1 zucchini, sliced
- 1 red bell pepper, diced
- 1 small red onion, thinly sliced
- 2 tablespoons olive oil
- Salt and pepper to taste
- 1/4 cup fresh basil, chopped
- 2 tablespoons balsamic vinegar
- 1/4 cup crumbled feta cheese (optional)

Directions:

1. Preheat the oven to 400°F (200°C).
2. In a baking sheet, toss cherry tomatoes, zucchini slices, diced red bell pepper, and thinly sliced red onion with olive oil, salt, and pepper.
3. Roast the vegetables in the preheated oven for about 20-25 minutes or until they are tender and slightly caramelized.
4. In a large salad bowl, combine the cooked quinoa with the roasted vegetables.
5. Add fresh basil to the salad and toss gently.

6. Drizzle balsamic vinegar over the salad and toss again to coat evenly.

7. If desired, sprinkle crumbled feta cheese over the top for added flavor.

8. Adjust salt and pepper according to your taste preferences.

9. Serve the Quinoa and Roasted Vegetable Salad as a hearty and nutritious option!

Cucumber and Chickpea Salad with Lemon Herb Dressing

Ingredients:

- 2 cucumbers, peeled and diced
- 1 can (15 oz) chickpeas, drained and rinsed
- 1 cup cherry tomatoes, halved
- 1/4 cup red bell pepper, finely chopped
- 1/4 cup fresh parsley, chopped
- 1/4 cup red onion, finely diced

For the Lemon Herb Dressing:

- 3 tablespoons olive oil
- Juice of 1 lemon
- 1 teaspoon Dijon mustard
- 1 clove garlic, minced
- 1 teaspoon dried oregano

- Salt and pepper to taste

Directions:

1. In a large salad bowl, combine diced cucumbers, chickpeas, cherry tomatoes, red bell pepper, fresh parsley, and diced red onion.

2. In a small bowl, whisk together olive oil, lemon juice, Dijon mustard, minced garlic, dried oregano, salt, and pepper to create the Lemon Herb Dressing.

3. Drizzle the dressing over the salad and toss gently until all ingredients are well coated.

4. Adjust the salt and pepper according to your taste preferences.

5. Allow the Cucumber and Chickpea Salad to chill in the refrigerator for about 15 minutes before serving.

6. Serve the salad as a light and protein-packed option!

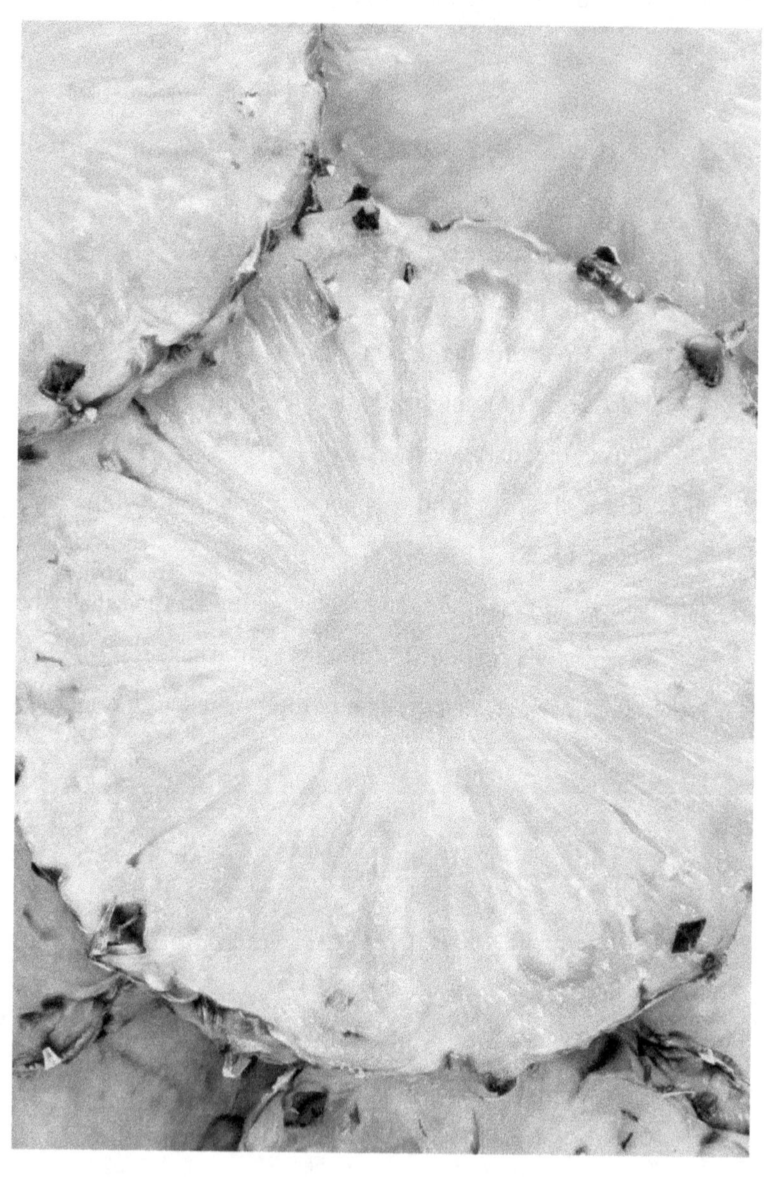

CHAPTER 9: SMOOTHIES

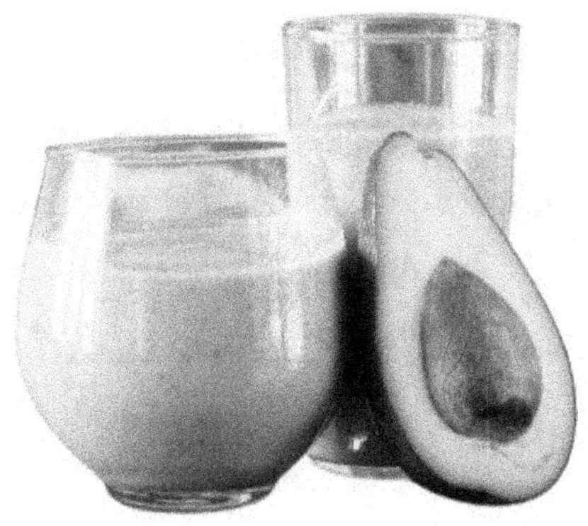

Citrus Avocado Smoothie

Ingredients:

- 1/2 avocado, peeled and pitted
- 1/2 cup pineapple chunks
- 1/2 orange, peeled and segmented
- 1 tablespoon fresh mint leaves
- 1 tablespoon flaxseeds
- 1/2 cup coconut water (unsweetened)

Directions:

1. In a blender, combine avocado, pineapple chunks, orange segments, fresh mint leaves, and flaxseeds.

2. Pour coconut water into the blender.

3. Blend on high speed until the mixture is smooth and creamy.

4. Check the consistency, and if needed, add more coconut water to achieve your desired thickness.

5. Pour the Citrus Avocado Smoothie into a glass, garnish with a mint sprig if desired, and enjoy immediately.

Turmeric Pineapple Bliss Smoothie

Ingredients:

- 1/2 cup pineapple chunks
- 1/2 cup cucumber, peeled and sliced
- 1/2 teaspoon turmeric powder
- 1/2 teaspoon grated ginger
- 1 tablespoon chia seeds
- 1/2 cup coconut water (unsweetened)
- Ice cubes (optional)

Directions:

1. In a blender, combine pineapple chunks, sliced cucumber, turmeric powder, grated ginger, and chia seeds.

2. Pour coconut water into the blender.

3. Add ice cubes if you prefer a colder smoothie.

4. Blend on high speed until the mixture is smooth and well combined.

5. Adjust the consistency by adding more coconut water if needed.

6. Pour the Turmeric Pineapple Bliss Smoothie into a glass, and savor the refreshing flavors.

Berry Almond Protein Smoothie

Ingredients:

- 1/2 cup mixed berries (blueberries, raspberries, strawberries)
- 1/4 cup almonds, soaked and peeled
- 1/2 banana
- 1 tablespoon almond butter
- 1/2 cup almond milk (unsweetened)
- 1 scoop pea protein powder
- Ice cubes (optional)

Directions:

1. In a blender, combine mixed berries, soaked and peeled almonds, banana, almond butter, and pea protein powder.

2. Pour almond milk into the blender.

3. Add ice cubes if you prefer a colder smoothie.

4. Blend on high speed until the mixture is smooth and creamy.

5. Adjust the thickness by adding more almond milk if desired.

6. Pour the Berry Almond Protein Smoothie into a glass, and enjoy this protein-packed, nutrient-rich treat.

Coconut Kale Green Smoothie

Ingredients:

- 1/2 cup kale leaves, stems removed
- 1/2 cup pineapple chunks
- 1/2 ripe avocado, peeled and pitted
- 1 tablespoon shredded coconut
- 1/2 lime, juiced
- 1/2 cup coconut water (unsweetened)
- Ice cubes (optional)

Directions:

1. In a blender, combine kale leaves, pineapple chunks, ripe avocado, shredded coconut, and lime juice.
2. Pour coconut water into the blender.
3. Add ice cubes if you prefer a colder smoothie.
4. Blend on high speed until the mixture is smooth and creamy.
5. Check the consistency and adjust with more coconut water if needed.
6. Pour the Coconut Kale Green Smoothie into a glass, and relish the tropical goodness.

Minty Melon Cucumber Smoothie

Ingredients:

- 1 cup honeydew melon, cubed
- 1/2 cucumber, peeled and sliced
- Handful of fresh mint leaves
- 1/2 lime, juiced
- 1 tablespoon flaxseeds
- 1/2 cup water or coconut water (unsweetened)
- Ice cubes (optional)

Directions:

1. In a blender, combine honeydew melon cubes, sliced cucumber, fresh mint leaves, lime juice, and flaxseeds.
2. Pour water or coconut water into the blender.
3. Add ice cubes if you prefer a colder smoothie.
4. Blend on high speed until the mixture is smooth and refreshing.
5. Adjust the thickness by adding more water or coconut water if needed.
6. Pour the Minty Melon Cucumber Smoothie into a glass, and enjoy the cool, mint-infused flavors.

Pomegranate Ginger Citrus Smoothie

Ingredients:

- 1/2 cup pomegranate seeds
- 1 orange, peeled and segmented
- 1/2 inch fresh ginger, peeled and grated
- 1/2 banana
- 1 tablespoon hemp seeds
- 1/2 cup water or almond milk (unsweetened)
- Ice cubes (optional)

Directions:

1. In a blender, combine pomegranate seeds, orange segments, grated ginger, banana, and hemp seeds.
2. Pour water or almond milk into the blender.
3. Add ice cubes if you prefer a colder smoothie.
4. Blend on high speed until the mixture is smooth and bursting with flavors.
5. Adjust the consistency by adding more water or almond milk if desired.
6. Pour the Pomegranate Ginger Citrus Smoothie into a glass, and relish the zesty and antioxidant-rich blend.

Berry Basil Bliss Smoothie

Ingredients:

- 1/2 cup mixed berries (blueberries, raspberries, strawberries)
- 4-5 fresh basil leaves
- 1/2 pear, cored and sliced
- 1 tablespoon chia seeds
- 1/2 cup green tea, cooled
- Ice cubes (optional)

Directions:

1. In a blender, combine mixed berries, fresh basil leaves, sliced pear, and chia seeds.
2. Pour cooled green tea into the blender.
3. Add ice cubes if you prefer a colder smoothie.
4. Blend on high speed until the mixture is smooth and bursting with fruity and herbal flavors.
5. Adjust the thickness by adding more green tea if needed.
6. Pour the Berry Basil Bliss Smoothie into a glass, and savor the delightful blend of berries and basil.

Coconut Pineapple Kale Smoothie

Ingredients:

- 1/2 cup pineapple chunks

- 1/2 cup kale leaves, stems removed
- 1/2 banana
- 2 tablespoons shredded coconut
- 1 tablespoon flaxseeds
- 1/2 cup coconut water
- Ice cubes (optional)

Directions:

1. In a blender, combine pineapple chunks, kale leaves, banana, shredded coconut, and flaxseeds.
2. Pour coconut water into the blender.
3. Add ice cubes if you prefer a colder smoothie.
4. Blend on high speed until the mixture is smooth and showcases the tropical flavors.
5. Adjust the consistency by adding more coconut water if desired.
6. Pour the Coconut Pineapple Kale Smoothie into a glass, and relish the delightful blend of coconut, pineapple, and nutrient-packed kale.

Mango Turmeric Sunshine Smoothie

Ingredients:

- 1/2 cup fresh mango chunks
- 1/2 teaspoon ground turmeric
- 1/2 cup cucumber, peeled and diced

- 1/2 lime, juiced

- 1 tablespoon honey

- 1/2 cup almond milk (unsweetened)

- Ice cubes (optional)

Directions:

1. In a blender, combine fresh mango chunks, ground turmeric, diced cucumber, lime juice, and honey.

2. Pour almond milk into the blender.

3. Add ice cubes if you prefer a colder smoothie.

4. Blend on high speed until the mixture is smooth and radiates the tropical flavors.

5. Adjust the sweetness with more honey if needed.

6. Pour the Mango Turmeric Sunshine Smoothie into a glass, and savor the fusion of mango, turmeric, and citrusy goodness.

Blueberry Mint Refresher Smoothie

Ingredients:

- 1/2 cup blueberries (fresh or frozen)

- 1/4 cup fresh mint leaves

- 1/2 apple, cored and chopped

- 1 tablespoon hemp seeds

- 1/2 cup coconut water

- 1/2 teaspoon spirulina powder (optional)

- Ice cubes (optional)

Directions:

1. In a blender, combine blueberries, fresh mint leaves, chopped apple, hemp seeds, and spirulina powder if using.
2. Pour coconut water into the blender.
3. Add ice cubes if you prefer a colder smoothie.
4. Blend on high speed until the mixture is smooth, and the mint imparts a refreshing aroma.
5. Adjust the thickness with more coconut water if desired.
6. Pour the Blueberry Mint Refresher Smoothie into a glass, and enjoy the unique blend of blueberries and mint.

Kiwi Basil Bliss Smoothie

Ingredients:

- 2 kiwis, peeled and sliced
- 1/2 banana
- 1/4 cup fresh basil leaves
- 1 tablespoon flaxseeds
- 1/2 cup coconut water
- 1/2 cup spinach leaves (optional for added nutrients)
- Ice cubes (optional)

Directions:

1. In a blender, combine kiwi slices, banana, fresh basil leaves, flaxseeds, and spinach if using.
2. Pour coconut water into the blender.
3. Add ice cubes if you prefer a colder smoothie.
4. Blend on high speed until the mixture is smooth, and the basil imparts a unique herbal note.
5. Adjust the sweetness by adding more banana if desired.
6. Pour the Kiwi Basil Bliss Smoothie into a glass, and savor the fusion of kiwi and basil.

Mango Mint Marvel Smoothie

Ingredients:

- 1 cup ripe mango, diced
- 1/2 cup cucumber, peeled and sliced
- 1/4 cup fresh mint leaves
- 1 tablespoon hemp seeds
- 1/2 cup almond milk
- 1/2 cup coconut water
- Ice cubes (optional)

Directions:

1. In a blender, combine diced mango, cucumber slices, fresh mint leaves, and hemp seeds.
2. Pour almond milk and coconut water into the blender.

3. Add ice cubes if you prefer a colder smoothie.

4. Blend on high speed until the mixture is smooth, and the mint adds a burst of freshness.

5. Adjust the sweetness by adding more mango if needed.

6. Pour the Mango Mint Marvel Smoothie into a glass, and relish the tropical and minty fusion.

Pineapple Kale Harmony Smoothie

Ingredients:

- 1 cup fresh pineapple chunks
- 1 cup kale, stems removed
- 1/2 banana
- 1 tablespoon flaxseeds
- 1/2 cup coconut water
- 1/2 cup water
- Ice cubes (optional)

Directions:

1. In a blender, combine fresh pineapple chunks, kale leaves, banana, and flaxseeds.
2. Pour coconut water and water into the blender.
3. Add ice cubes if you prefer a colder smoothie.
4. Blend on high speed until the mixture is smooth, and the kale adds a nutritional boost.
5. Adjust the sweetness by adding more bananas if needed.
6. Pour the Pineapple Kale Harmony Smoothie into a glass, and savor the tropical-kale fusion.

CONCLUSION

In conclusion, this Blood Type A Diet Cookbook emphasizes the significance of adopting a tailored approach to eating for maximum health and wellbeing. By adapting recipes to the specific requirements of people with Blood Type A, this cookbook strives to empower readers to make educated and aware nutritional choices.

Throughout these pages, we've looked at a selection of tasty and nutrient-dense meals that have been carefully chosen to follow the Blood Type A diet principles. From vivid salads to filling main meals, each dish has been designed with the nutritional needs of Blood Type A people in mind, encouraging a healthy relationship between food and body.

Remember that the Blood Type A diet is more than simply a collection of recipes; it is a lifestyle choice that highlights the relationship between your blood type and the things you eat. As you embark on this culinary adventure, consider how these dishes may be smoothly integrated into your everyday life, benefiting not just your physical well-being but also promoting a conscious and holistic approach to health.

Finally, we advise you to embrace the benefits of eating according to your blood type. Nourishing your body with the appropriate nutrients will significantly improve your overall health and energy levels. We hope this cookbook is a beneficial resource on your journey to attaining and sustaining optimum health, laying the groundwork for a lifestyle that values both nutrition and well-being.

Cheers to a healthier

and

happy you!

Weekly
Meal Plan

Week: ___________

	BREAKFAST	LUNCH	DINNER	SNACKS
MON				
TUE				
WED				
THU				
FRI				
SAT				
SUN				

Shopping list

___________ ___________

___________ ___________

___________ ___________

Notes:

Weekly
Meal Plan

Week: ___________

	BREAKFAST	LUNCH	DINNER	SNACKS
MON				
TUE				
WED				
THU				
FRI				
SAT				
SUN				

Shopping list

_______________ _______________

_______________ _______________

_______________ _______________

Notes:

Weekly
Meal Plan

Week:________

	BREAKFAST	LUNCH	DINNER	SNACKS
MON				
TUE				
WED				
THU				
FRI				
SAT				
SUN				

Shopping list

_____________ _____________

_____________ _____________

_____________ _____________

Notes:

Weekly
Meal Plan

Week: ______________

	BREAKFAST	LUNCH	DINNER	SNACKS
MON				
TUE				
WED				
THU				
FRI				
SAT				
SUN				

Shopping list

_______________ _______________

_______________ _______________

_______________ _______________

Notes:

Weekly
Meal Plan

Week: _____________

	BREAKFAST	LUNCH	DINNER	SNACKS
MON				
TUE				
WED				
THU				
FRI				
SAT				
SUN				

Shopping list

__________ __________

__________ __________

__________ __________

Notes:

Weekly
Meal Plan

Week:_____________

	BREAKFAST	LUNCH	DINNER	SNACKS
MON				
TUE				
WED				
THU				
FRI				
SAT				
SUN				

Shopping list

_________________   _________________

_________________   _________________

_________________   _________________

Notes:

Weekly
Meal Plan

Week:___________

	BREAKFAST	LUNCH	DINNER	SNACKS
MON				
TUE				
WED				
THU				
FRI				
SAT				
SUN				

Shopping list

_______________   _______________

_______________   _______________

_______________   _______________

Notes:

Weekly
Meal Plan

Week: ___________

	BREAKFAST	LUNCH	DINNER	SNACKS
MON				
TUE				
WED				
THU				
FRI				
SAT				
SUN				

Shopping list

___________ ___________

___________ ___________

___________ ___________

Notes:

Weekly
Meal Plan

Week: _______________

	BREAKFAST	LUNCH	DINNER	SNACKS
MON				
TUE				
WED				
THU				
FRI				
SAT				
SUN				

Shopping list

_______________ _______________

_______________ _______________

_______________ _______________

Notes:

Weekly
Meal Plan

Week: ___________

	BREAKFAST	LUNCH	DINNER	SNACKS
MON				
TUE				
WED				
THU				
FRI				
SAT				
SUN				

Shopping list

_____________ _____________

_____________ _____________

_____________ _____________

Notes: